Your Seco

Rising Above the Myths of Aging

Live ~Learn ~Laugh ~Love ~Lead

YOUR SECOND FIFTY

Rising Above the Myths of Aging

FRANK MOFFATT
with Michael Roach

YSF Industries

Your Second Fifty
Rising Above the Myths of Aging!
Written by Frank Moffatt
With Michael Roach
Copyright © 2009
By Frank Moffatt
With Michael Roach
Second Edition
Published by YSF INDUSTRIES
Calgary, Canada
www.yoursecondfifty.com
info@yoursecondfifty.com

ISBN: 978-0-9865568-5-2

Health, Fitness & Dieting – Aging

Artwork – Diane Martin – www.mypagedesigner.com

What others are saying:

Frank and I have been friends for close to 15 years. The fire and passion that he brings to every project will leave you feeling rest assured that he has left no stone unturned when it comes to what is important in living "your second fifty" to its fullest. This book is an excellent introduction for all of us who have entered our second fifty, opening doors and giving us direction on how to maximize the remainder of our life.
Neil Thompson, Deputy Managing Director, BEC Tero Entertainment PLC, Bangkok, Thailand

Your Second Fifty certainly looks like a wealth of information and knowledge for those looking to live an enriched, rewarding second half of their life.
The late Harley Hotchkiss, Chairman of the board of the National Hockey League, Companions of the Order of Canada.

Often in life we become trapped by beliefs that we have acquired from family, friends and piers. Certainly their intention wasn't negative, but in many cases their beliefs simply weren't true. In Your Second Fifty, Frank addresses many of these inaccurate beliefs and provides you with positive truths that will guide you to an amazing second fifty.
Peggy McColl, New York Times Best Selling Author, International Speaker and Mentor

My fiftieth birthday was a wake-up call. Creating balance, fulfillment and a greater security for myself and my family, while always important, quickly became a priority. Reading 'Your Second Fifty' provided me with the tools to understand and create a well-rounded approach to my Mental, Emotional, Physical, Financial and Spiritual dimensions. Thanks Frank, for providing the avenue to help me, and many others, identify and understand both our 'why' and 'how' and to live our second fifty with purpose and fulfillment.
Geoffrey Foster, VP Taco Time Canad

I'm a firm believer in the quote "There are three types of people in this world: those who make things happen, those who watch things happen and those who wonder what happened." When Frank sets his sights on something there's no question, he will make things happen. In his book Your Second Fifty, Frank outlines the fears and myths that at times can stop us from making things happen and provides us with the steps necessary to alter these limiting beliefs.
Mike Sotski, President Sunridge RV, Calgary, Alberta, Canada

From the moment I met Frank I knew that I had met one of the most influential people I have had the pleasure to know and call my friend. Frank has the profound ability to draw on life's many humorous and profound stories to create a tapestry of lessons that make one's evolution in life a simple and fun journey to explore. This book is for anyone, as it draws on the wisdom of the ages to be enjoyed at any point in one's life journey. You and I are both so incredibly fortunate to hold this book in our hands, and to take it with us into the next decades of our lives."
Lars Gustafsson, Founder of The BodyMind Institute, Calgary, Alberta, Canada

As a personal trainer and fitness instructor, I'm very aware of the importance of maintaining a healthy body throughout our life and especially once we've entered our second fifty. I believe that age is just a number and getting older doesn't mean that we have to stop being active and doing the things we love. I also believe that it's never too late to start! Rather than letting age impact our outlook on life, I believe a positive attitude is what really makes the difference. In Frank's book not only does he provide a solid basic understanding of the importance of health, but he clearly explains the importance of balancing all of our dimensions, Mental, Emotional, Physical, Financial and Spiritual. If you wish to invest in "your second fifty" a great place to start would be this book.
Jari Love, Certified Personal Trainer and the Creator of Get RIPPED!™ Workout DVD Series

I had the privilege of working with Frank in Thailand on a project near and dear to his heart, the making of a record by two of his boys Clint and Bob. The experience enriched me immensely as I witnessed the blossoming of a man who had scaled the heights and delved the depths of the music business, yet had the humility and humanity to reach within and seek the wisdom which eludes most of us in life. Although I'm still in my first fifty, "Your Second Fifty" inspires me to do what Frank has done so well, and that's simply to embrace life and live it, no matter what your age.
Gerald V. Dibbayawan, Chief Executive Officer – TGV Cinemas Sdn Bhd (Malaysia)

Frank Moffatt's "Your Second Fifty" is an encouraging and amazing book that offers insight into untapped skills and talents that may not be utilized. "Your Second Fifty" does not take the cookie cutter approach of offering simple advice, but offers an opportunity to realize and motivate people to make changes they want in all areas of life. Frank has emulated the principles put forth in his book and continues enhance

his own experience within his own second fifty. He willingly shares with anyone on the quest who has realized there are no limits to what can be achieved in the second stage of life.
Bob Steeg, Addictions Counsellor, Biggar, Saskatchewan, Canada

It's refreshing to learn from Franks book "Your Second Fifty" that for those of us who have reached this 'ripe old age', and sometimes fear or are apprehensive about what potentially lies ahead, should fear no more, and should take his advice, stay active, be creative and live life to the fullest, as there is still so much we can look forward to, and achieve, with the right mind-set and positive attitude.
Nigel Peters, Director, Midas Promotions, Bahrain, Hong Kong, Singapore and Manila Philippines

I was blessed to play in over 1,300 games in the NHL and over that period of time I watched many talented players come and go. The key to succeeding as I saw it was the ability to adjust and adapt to an ever changing game. In "Your Second Fifty" Frank provides his readers with the tools required to positively adjust and adapt to the ever changing challenges of life over fifty.
Dave Babych, NHL All-star, Vancouver Canucks

Each day we're provided with new information that reveals our unlimited potential as human beings. In "Your Second Fifty" you'll be introduced to a number of ways in which you can make changes to enhance each of your five dimensions and develop behaviors that will embrace this true potential. As we age we owe it ourselves to remain open and flexible and with Frank's guidance your second fifty has every opportunity to be a lot better than your first fifty!
Ronny Gozali, President, Catur Mitra Adhikara, pt, Jakarta, Indonesia

My name is Jeff and I'm a Workaholic... Frank has written a book that has the potential to improve the lives of millions of people that likely don't even realize their lives could be improved. Far to often we work until we retire and then the question is "What now?" In Your Second Fifty the "What now?" is spelled out for you in an easy to follow process that continually opens doors to a more positive, productive way of life. "Thank" you Frank. "Thank" you for reminding me I'm turning 50 next year. "Thank" you for reminding me that that word "thank" could become a euphemism for a word I can't say in front of my two year old daughter.
Jeffrey R.W. Rath, B.A. (Hons.), LL.B. (Hons.), Barrister & Solicitor, Rath & Company, Calgary, Canada

Frank Moffatt is a lightning rod of passion and is on a mission to inspire others to live to the fullest. Frank's words come crackling off the page in his new book, "Your Second Fifty" -- and it is what is needed when it comes to direction and guidance for those who want to make the best of the rest of their lives.

Kelly Sullivan Walden, "Doctor Dream"- Bestselling author, It's All In Your Dreams

If there's one thing I know about my Dad it's that he has unbelievable passion for helping others. That passion gave him the ability to immerse himself in the writing of this book. Now I may not be in my second fifty yet, BUT that being said, there is a wealth of information in this book that I can use in my life today! Your life starts whenever you decide it does, and this book gives you many ideas to help you discover fresh ways to look at life. It's worth every penny because you are!

Bob Moffatt, International Recording Artist, Songwriter and Producer, Nashville, TN

I think I speak for a lot of us in our second fifty when I say, we know we're going to live longer, what we want to do, is live those years happier and healthier. In Frank's book "Your Second Fifty" he gives us a nice outline of the areas we need to work on and what to do to give us that opportunity. Again for most of us it's not a question of whether we want to do it - the question is - how do we do it?

Robert W. McMahon, Director, Rohn Products International, USA, Saudi Arabia and S.E. Asia

Frank and I have been friends for some time now and have many things in common, some pleasant – writing books and looking for ways to make the world a better place, some challenging – assisting loved one's face their greatest challenges. As you enter "your second fifty" it never hurts to have a coach, especially one that has your best interests at heart!

Robert Urbanowski, Best Selling Author of "Kickback", President Guru Marketing

I've interviewed more than 400 top achievers around the world, and without a doubt, Frank is one of these achievers. "Your second Fifty" is a great read, filled with Frank's knowledge and experiences. This book would be prefect for anyone looking to create more or better results in their lives.

Douglas Vermeeren, The Gratitude Experiment, Author, Speaker, Calgary, Alberta, Canada

Foreword

by Dan Botha MD

A S A MEDICAL practitioner that specializes in mature adult care, I'm amazed at all the new medical discoveries that possess the potential to extend a person's life. Although extending a person's life is great, living that life positively and productively for their remaining years is far more important.

Enter my good friend **Frank Moffatt** – who has written this wonderful, simple-to-follow instruction manual outlining how to live your "second fifty" positively and productively. In this empowering book, you will discover your five dimensions and how to find balance within them.

To live a well-balanced life, we need all of our dimensions functioning at a high level – mentally, emotionally, physically, financially and spiritually. Throughout the journey of *Your Second Fifty*, Frank will both entertain you and guide you through these dimensions. You will become aware, possibly for the first time, of your potential and how much you really have left to enjoy and share with others.

Far too often we subconsciously allow myths and limiting beliefs to stop us from being all we can be. In *Your Second Fifty*, Frank tackles these myths head on and walks you through the steps to take that will not only extend your life, but that will allow you to maximize each remaining day of your life on earth.

Frank is a loving, inspirational coach and dedicated teacher. He brings immense passion to every challenge he embraces, including this book you're reading right now. *Your Second Fifty* opens the door to your potential, a new way of life, and an opportunity to live your life to the fullest.

I know that when you start reading and living *Your Second Fifty*, your life will never be the same. You will become more aware of exactly who you are, what you are capable of doing and how to productively spend the rest of your life.

Enjoy your journey through *Your Second Fifty*. Learn all you can and be all you can be. In reading this book, you've taken the first step. Continue taking action to make these simple adjustments in your life and you will be doing your part in making our world a better place.

Wishing you a wonderful second fifty!

Dan Botha MD, MBChB , MBA
www.drbotha.com

Frank's Thanks!

People can only learn when their original assumptions have been broken.
Steve Chang – Founder, Trend Micro

YOUR SECOND FIFTY is a collaboration of hundreds of people, their writings, their wisdom and their courage to question previously held beliefs and to look positively and progressively into the future. I sincerely hope that these efforts will lead you to explore your own unlimited potentialities – and to come to the realization that given the time and effort, a fantastic and fulfilling second fifty years is well within your control. To all of you that have inspired me and shown me the path to my unlimited potential, I say thank you.

To Michael Pond – Thank you for your inspiration, ideas and guidance pertaining to the layout of *Your Second Fifty*, for your feedback on various chapters, for providing me with a quality writing environment and for offering me employment – which allowed me to continue to write while covering my basic needs and expenses. Without your help this book would not have become a reality.

To Dale Wallace – You are the man! Editing my run-on sentences so that the readers wouldn't be hyperventilating by the second chapter is an amazing feat in of itself. But to assist me to orchestrate all of these little snippets of information into that of a book, now that's something - wow!

To Michael Roach – You provide the wild entrepreneur in me with a necessary sense of balance. Your vision in seeing where we can take *Your Second Fifty* and all the people that we can help is a blessing to us all.

To my sons, thank you for your unconditional love and support. You are truly amazing young men; you have taught me so much. I wish you well as you continue to blaze your own paths throughout your journeys. To my family and friends, thank you for your spiritual guidance, wisdom and diversity in acceptance, compassion and understanding.

In the words of Alan Cohen:
It takes a lot of courage to release the familiar and seemingly secure, to embrace the new. But there is no real security in what is no longer meaningful. There is more security in the adventurous and exciting, for in movement there is life, and in change there is power.

Special Thanks

To Yunia Astuti, Ronny Gonzali, Bob McMahon, Sandip Roy, Mike Sotski, Harley Hotchkiss, Helen Roach, Tanwita Roy, Bill Moffatt, Neil Thompson, The Bangkok Boys, Peggy McColl, Jari Love, Tony Ma, Andrew Biggs, Grace Celeste, Lars Gustafsson, Gerald Dibbayawan, Dennis Huntley, Komalrat Maksaman, Mom and Dad, Geoff Foster, Nigel Peters, Raksit Rakkandee, T. Harv Eker, Doug Vermeeren, Prapaichit Potpan, Patcharee Poo-sommai, Diane Martin, the Gramedia Team (Indra, Pauline, Lucia). This book couldn't and wouldn't have been completed without your help and the help of others. If I missed you I'm sorry – keep in mind that these are only words on paper and my true gratitude for your kindness is in my heart!

Michael's Thanks!

TO MY BEAUTIFUL wife, Helen – You've spent your nursing career providing loving care for people in elderly care residences. Along with sharing with me a wealth of experience of the various mindsets that develop with aging, you've extended to me a great deal of patience and understanding while I worked on this project. Thank you!

To Frank – Thank you for allowing me to stand on your shoulders and envision the possibilities that exist. Your personal motto of "Keep smiling!" and your passion to help others is a blessing and inspiration to all. I enjoy being a witness to the positive legacy you're building in this world.

To Lars Gustafsson – As my nutritionist, life coach & spiritual teacher during the past few years, you've offered me a wonderful new outlook of our world, on so many levels. You are an amazing soul.

To my wonderful children – you are the greatest inspiration behind everything I do. I love you immensely.

Table of Contents

Introduction

I could not, at any age, be content to take my place by the fireside and simply look on. Life was meant to be lived. Curiosity must be kept alive. One must never, for whatever reason, turn his back on life.
Eleanor Roosevelt

A T AGE 95, Nola Ochs became the world's oldest college graduate. At age 100 Fauja Singh completed the Toronto Waterfront Marathon in just over 8 hours. Jeanne Calment of France died at 122 years of age. Nerve cells in the human brain and muscle cells in the heart have the capacity to last more than 100 years. So why do our bodies break down and the majority of us die well before we reach 100 years of age? Because most of us believe that's just the way it is supposed to be.

Throughout *Your Second Fifty*, we intend to challenge **traditional** beliefs and present you with an alternative way of thinking. The information provided is only a guide – the journey is yours. We believe that when our mental, emotional, physical, financial and spiritual dimensions are in balance, a long and healthy, productive second fifty years is unquestionably within our reach.

In *Your Second Fifty*, we will help open the endless possibilities that lay before you. We do not intend to lecture or preach. Instead, we will simply and humbly offer a path through the five dimensions of your life: the mental, emotional, physical, financial and spiritual. It is essential to understand that before you begin this journey, you must be prepared to challenge old beliefs and explore new possibilities. If you are willing to have an open mind, you will discover within you the capacity to completely change your own experience of aging.

Life can sometimes seem like an endless series of challenges and hurdles. The key to successfully addressing and confronting those challenges is *discipline*. The manner in which you address your challenges will determine the degree of your successes or failures. Anyone who truly desires to experience true success must also accept that *persistence* is a natural part of living and a key component in overcoming life's challenges. This newly attained wisdom will serve you well as you continue to apply self-discipline to life's ongoing journey. Know that your life is in your hands and you are ultimately responsible for it in every way.

Society has become geared for the quick fix, heaping great praise and expectations on the experts that proclaim, "I know your problem – here's the magic pill!" Nothing could be further from the truth when attempting life changes. These experts don't change us – we change ourselves. We change ourselves by accepting, surrendering, and then taking corrective action.

> *Half our life is spent trying to find something to do with the time we have*
> *rushed through life trying to save.*
> **Will Rogers**

Our mental, emotional, physical, financial and spiritual lives are intricately linked. When one or more of these areas are ignored, the holistic result (our self) is out of balance and lacks cohesion. To use an analogy, if one tire on a car is low of air pressure and out of balance, the subsequent poor performance of that tire directly influences the overall performance of the entire vehicle. Or, for example if a woman were to train five hours a week in the gym with aspirations of shapely hips and legs, but perceived herself with a pear shaped figure, she would be pretty much guaranteed little chance of attaining her physical goals.

Thus we need to positively align our mental capacities, emotional states, spiritual practices and financial beliefs with our physical goals, for our full potential to be realized.

Question Your Thinking

> *A few years back, three generations of women and their families*
> *gathered for Christmas Eve. It was their tradition to fix a large*
> *ham for dinner and this year it was the youngest woman's*
> *opportunity to cook the ham.*

> *As she had been taught by her mother, she got out her large*
> *roasting pan, sliced the back end off of the ham. Her young*
> *husband watched and admired as she prepared the ham. But he*
> *was a bit confused as to why she had cut off the back end of the*

ham, so he asked and she replied, "That's the way my mother always did it."

So the young man went to his Mother-In-Law and asked her why she always cut the end off the ham before cooking it. "Well son, she said, that is how mother taught me to do it.

The young husband then decided to then ask his wife's grandmother the same question.

So he approached the elderly grandmother. "Granny," he uttered respectfully, "Why do all the women in your family cut the back end off of the ham before cooking it?"

"Son," she replied as she sat up in her wheel chair, "I don't have a clue as to why those silly girls do that. As for me, when I was a young bride I didn't have a pan big enough to hold a whole ham so I cut the end off to make it fit."

When our ideas and decisions are based upon myths and folklore, we run the risk of limiting our true potential. Unfortunately, in many cases, people are far too willing to accept information if a trusted person tells them.

We have always been taught that aging is irreversible and that a progressive decline in our mental, emotional, and physical capacities is a natural process. Nonsense. In *Your Second Fifty* we encourage you to change the way you think about aging – and experience for yourself the beautiful reality of a revitalized and rejuvenated self.

Deepak Chopra says that our minds have been conditioned to believe that the normal experience of the body and its aging is a habit of our thinking and behavior, and that by changing how we think and behave, we can actually change our minds and our body's experience of aging.

Harvard psychologist, Ellen Langer, took groups of men in their seventies and eighties who were encouraged to behave and think as if they were twenty years younger. These men showed definite physical changes of much younger men after only five days. Thus, if we have the mental and emotional expectation that we are younger, we have a far greater opportunity to live longer than the norm is expected.

In the book *BioMarkers* by William Evans, researchers have medically proven that the body is constantly rebuilding itself and can actually grow *younger* with the right conditions. So the reality is that if you are willing to change your way of thinking, your emotional states, your physical fitness, your financial stability and your spiritual practices, then your body and mind will have a much improved opportunity for regeneration, renewal, and revitalization.

Quantum physics theory* compels us to change how we view the whole process of life, the human body, and aging. It suggests that our essence, or who we really are, is beyond the mental and physical realms, as we know them. That is, from the perspective of quantum physics, the spiritual realm of existence is the cornerstone for improving our mental, physical and emotional health. The spiritual domain is the true source of our happiness, freedom, joy, and sense of fulfillment and our financial stability helps to reduce stress and provides us with an opportunity to seek out a healthier lifestyle. Quantum physicists herald that we all have the capacity to alter our physical body and the functioning of our minds. Some scientists now believe that we can determine and change the biological age and physiological condition in which we want our body and mind to be.

> ** Quantum physics is a branch of science that deals with discrete, indivisible units of energy called quanta as described by the Quantum Theory. Quantum theory is the theoretical basis of modern physics that explains the nature and behavior of matter and energy on the atomic and subatomic level.*

Now some of these ideas may be difficult for you to accept. However, for you to grow mentally, emotionally, physically, financially and spiritually, you must be willing to consider new research that disproves previously accepted beliefs, based upon folklore, myths, and outdated research. These concepts are new and challenging, but within our reach if we can discard the naysayers' comments and believe in our potential. The Wright Brothers believed in possibilities and flight became a reality. It all comes down to personal faith in our ability to succeed in what we believe.

Live your life, forget your age.
Norman Vincent Peale

To better understand and accept this new way of thinking, it's important to understand the three types of age classifications and how age is categorized. These classifications include the following: chronological age, biological age and psychological age.

> ***Chronological age*** *is the number of years that have passed in our lives starting from the date of our birth and the subsequent passage of time according to the annual calendar. This age cannot be changed. Ironically, chronological age is the least significant factor in determining how old we feel or function.*

> ***Biological age*** *is the measure of how well our physiological systems are functioning. Our biological age is calculated through biological markers; some of which include body fat composition, cholesterol levels, blood pressure, aerobic functioning, and bone density. As expected, our biological age can be the same as or differ significantly from our chronological age. In other words, an individual who is chronologically fifty years of age can be functioning biologically at a much younger age or a much older age, depending on the way they live their life. People who take care of themselves can have a younger biological age; whereas, an individual who is sedentary and has poor eating habits can have an older biological age.*

> ***Psychological age*** *is our own personal experience of how old we feel. So if we tap into the energy that determines how old we feel our body can actually become younger by utilizing different mental capacities. Thus, how we think we feel can actually determine how young or old we are. The most significant factor in determining how old we actually feel and function is our <u>attitude</u>. This attitude translates into the saying "growing older means growing better." If we believe and expect our mental and physical capacities to diminish with age, they probably will. On the other hand, if we believe and expect that we can attain youthful vitality; our experience will most likely follow that course of thought.*

Michael Pond R.P.N., M.S.W.

Hopefully by now your interest has been piqued and you have come to the conclusion, "What do I have to lose, by giving this a try?" The answer, "Nothing but a little fear-based comfort!" However, that little fear actually has the capacity to completely immobilize us. So how do we overcome that fear? The answer is by self-discipline. By self-disciple we are referring to our ability to apply our willpower over the execution and completion of a given task, even though we would rather be doing something else.

Then we need to set attainable goals that we are comfortable with, and goals that will provide us with long term, lasting results. Once we have a solid understanding of discipline and goals we can begin the process of exploring the countless opportunities of enhancing our five dimensions.

Our Five Dimensions

The first dimension we will explore and learn to enhance is our **Mental Dimension**. Our Mental Dimension encompasses all aspects of consciousness and intellect and is manifested through any combination of thought, imagination, perception, memory, or will. In other words, our Mental Dimension provides us with the capability to reason – the unaided ability to form concepts, to analyze, or to study. By shifting our Mental Dimension alone, we can completely change our lives – and this does include our memory.

The second dimension we will address is our **Emotional Dimension**. Our Emotional Dimension encompasses our ability, skill, or capacity to assess, perceive, and manage our emotions. It is our own experience of our feelings and what we do with those feelings that is the manifestation of how we perceive ourselves and how others perceive us.

The third dimension covered will be our **Physical Dimension**. Our Physical Dimension pertains to our material being and bodily functions. These components encompass not only our aerobic fitness, our muscle strength/endurance, and our flexibility, but also our nutrition, diet, and how we effectively care for our bodies.

The fourth dimension is our **Financial Dimension**. Our Financial Dimension relates to our values and beliefs pertaining to money. Do we allow it to enter our life, do we push it away, do we manage it correctly and do we help others?

The fifth dimension is our **Spiritual Dimension**. Our Spiritual Dimension relates to our faith and beliefs, our willingness to accept a higher power, our commitment to an honorable value system, and the laws of nature. This dimension, for some of us, can be the most difficult to accept and understand, yet it is the most significant and powerful dimension of the five.

In *Your Second Fifty*, we will give you a fifty-day program of activities and inspirational readings that will form a solid five-dimensional foundation for a second fifty years of youthful health and vigor.

Life is what we make of it. We've all had hard days, and everyone faces challenges and extreme difficulties throughout life. However, if we provide equal attention to all five dimensions in our life, each will act as a support system for the other and provide us with the complete internal strength necessary to not just continue, but thrive. Patiently and persistently, one step at a time, as each dimension grows stronger, all dimensions grow stronger, and the individual grows stronger too.

Persevere and you are bound to succeed. Thomas Edison said that perseverance is the secret to success. It took him thousands of trials to successfully invent the incandescent light bulb. It took George de Mestral eight years of trial and error until he developed a successful design for Velcro. As with all good things, success begins one step at a time, and before we know it something magical has happened.

It is my sincere wish that *Your Second Fifty* opens new doors and inspires you to challenge yourself and your unlimited capacity to live a healthy, balanced, and fulfilling second fifty years. So now let's get started, because today is the first day of the rest of your life and whatever happened in our past plays no role what-so-ever now or in our future.

> *Twenty years from now you will be more disappointed by the things you didn't do than by the ones you did do. So throw off the bowlines. Sail away from the safe harbor. Catch the trade winds in your sails. Explore. Dream. Discover.*
> **Mark Twain**

The Frank Experience – Introduction

I was fifty-three years old when I began writing *Your Second Fifty*. My age alone hardly makes me an expert at living to 100. However, after all the research that I've done, and with all those whom I've spoken that are happy and healthy and well into their second fifty, I'm absolutely convinced that with a little discipline and effort, the abundant rewards of a healthy, happy and balanced second fifty years are well within our reach.

Each of us starts on the same playing field and the only difference is our perceived view of ourselves and others. We don't have a disadvantage unless we are informed we have a disadvantage, and then accept and believe in this disadvantage in order to actualize the disadvantage. Great men and women weren't awarded their talents they are a product of their diligence, effort and it persistence. It isn't luck and it isn't chance. Success comes from hard, smart work and persistence.

Leonardo da Vinci, Albert Einstein and Bill Gates represent exceptional mental dimensions. Martin Luther King Jr., Mother Theresa and Nelson Mandela demonstrate extraordinary emotional control. Jesse Owens, Terry Fox and Wayne Gretzky illustrate astonishing physical dimensions, Warren Buffett, Bill Gates and Donald Trump exhibit astounding financial dimensions and The Buddha, Jesus of Nazareth and Muhammad exemplify profound spiritual dimensions. None of them attained their place in history because it was their God given right – they went out and lived their passion one day at a time and as with everything else in life – staying focused, putting in the time and living life to the best of their ability paid off in them actualizing their dreams.

So, is it important for each of us to become worldly renown as a great mind, a pillar in the face of adversity, a champion of champions, a money magnate or a worshiped spiritual figure? I think not, but I do believe it's important to challenge ourselves daily and to do everything in our power to be the best we can be. At the same time it's important to discipline ourselves to overcome our innately lazy tendencies to waste our only truly precious commodity – our time, and in turn, our lives.

You've got to live it – to live!
Frank Moffatt

Discipline

In reading the lives of great men, I found that the first victory they won was over themselves...self-discipline with all of them came first."
Harry S Truman

WHILE IT CERTAINLY does appear that our future looks exceeding bright, the road to attaining these rewards will be difficult and at times downright uncomfortable. So how will we overcome these difficulties? Discipline! Or more precisely, *self-discipline*. Self-discipline is the act of disciplining ourselves to do what it takes to have what we want, even though we would prefer to be doing something else, or nothing at all.

> *Life is difficult. This is a great truth; one of the greatest truths. It is a great truth because once we truly see this truth, we transcend it. Once we truly know that life is difficult – once we truly understand and accept it – then life is no longer difficult. Because once it is accepted, the fact that life is difficult no longer matters. **
> **Scott Peck**

> ** The first of the "Four Noble Truths" which Buddha taught was "Life is suffering."*

However, for most of us Peck's idea is almost impossible to accept because if we accept his idea, we are then compelled to accept that we are completely responsible for our own experience of life. Most people have difficulty accepting responsibility for the results of their choices and the decisions that they make. Instead, they prefer to believe that it is the actions of others that cause their pain and suffering. However, once they neglect or relegate to others (blame) the consequences of their choices; they no longer have to take responsibility. Without taking responsibility we can't effectively apply a solution to our perceived problem.

> *If you do not conquer self, you will be conquered by self.*
> **Napoleon Hill**

So how do we accept and apply self-discipline in our lives?

First, we must be willing to *delay gratification*. We need to eat our dinner before we eat our dessert. Complete the task at hand, no matter how challenging, before we take a break. We need to overcome our natural instinct to run from mental or physical pain.

Delaying gratification is becoming more and more of a challenge today because of the instantaneous gratification that marketing presents and the perception that there is a quick simple fix for everything. Computers can fix our grammar, talk show hosts have countless guests with quick fixes for all our emotions, plastic surgeons suck away our fat, and televangelists dissolve our misdeeds for the week with one quick outburst of words on Sunday morning.

We are conditioned to look for the quick fix for almost everything, because we want that immediate payoff. But the truth is everything that is important takes time and determination and while a quick fix gives us instantaneous gratification, without continued work, diligence and commitment, our misery is certain to find its way back. Sadly, the pain we were looking to eradicate has actually only been suppressed for the time being.

Second, we must be willing to *accept responsibility*. Accept that we are completely in control of how we respond and react to all the events in our lives. No one limits our ability to learn but ourselves. We may not learn as quickly as others, but if we put the time in we will most certainly learn whatever it is we are attempting to learn.

> *With self-discipline, most anything is possible.*
> **Theodore Roosevelt**

Third, we must be *dedicated to the truth*. This statement isn't easy because we've been trained to make excuses, justify, manipulate, and twist the truth to suit our needs. But truth is reality and anything unreal is then false. So anything that has not yet transpired can only be unreal and a figment of our imagination, concocted by our ego. If we are overweight, the truth is we ate more food than our body required

– it's that simple. (Thyroid Foundation of Canada states - The safest approach is lifestyle modification that results in decreased caloric intake by changing eating habits and increased expenditure of calories by exercising more. Even though weight control may be more difficult after being diagnosed with hypothyroidism, it is still quite possible.)

> *Self-respect is the fruit of discipline: the sense of dignity grows with the ability to say no to oneself.*
> **Abraham Heschel**

Finally, we must *live a life of balance*. Balance means we are willing to adjust to each situation, to remain flexible and to consider that not everything is possible all of the time. Highs make lows and lows make highs. If we want peace in our lives, we need to keep ourselves balanced.

> *Procrastination is the fear of success. People procrastinate because they are afraid of the success that they know will result if they move ahead now. Because success is heavy, carries a responsibility with it, it is much easier to procrastinate and live on the 'someday I'll' philosophy.*
> **Denis Waitley**

Initially, self-discipline may appear as a hardship full of pain and frustration, but the reality couldn't be anything further from the truth. Mastery of self-discipline not only leads us out of internal frustration and pain, but into genuine self-confidence and satisfaction. We are capable of achieving whatever we want, whenever we want, once we put our minds to it.

The Frank Experience - Discipline

For me discipline has always been a difficult hurdle because I'm always looking for the easiest, shortest, and quickest way out of every situation. Sadly, I'm usually trying with words and not actions. However, interestingly enough, everything that I've ever accomplished in my life is directly related to me asserting my will on a consistent basis and remaining focused on my primary goal, which in turn equals the act of self-discipline.

At 52, I decided I was going to run a marathon. For a guy that grew up with asthma and could barely make the four laps prior to a football practice, I don't know what came over me, to lead me to this crazy idea. But once it was in place, discipline not only became a requirement, but a necessity.

Every morning I got up at 6:00 am, put on my shorts, shirt, and runners and took off out the door. I began training by running one kilometer a day (although for the first couple of weeks half of the kilometer was spent walking). I despised the first hundred meters, but I told myself that it would get better. Because I didn't give in, because I never quit, and because I exerted some discipline, over time the training did indeed get easier.

By the end of the first month, I was up to three kilometers a day. My blisters had become calluses and my gut stopped jiggling so much – or should I say bouncing. During the second month I had moved up to five kilometers, twice a week. Though trust me, I was still counting every single step.

In the third month, I had pushed one of my weekly five kilometer runs up to eight kilometers, but was now taking two days off a week to recuperate. That's what I read in a training article, and who am I to argue with the professionals. In the fourth month, I was putting in a ten kilometer run every second Saturday. Some days everything just clicked – I actually felt like a runner!

During the fifth month, I did one twenty kilometer run – three weeks before the race. After that run I really questioned myself. Was I completely nuts? Twenty kilometers wasn't even half of what I needed to run to finish the marathon. I was nearly crawling by the end of the twenty kilometers. But on November 27, 2005 – down twelve kilograms from when I started – I crossed the finish line in 4:29:51, in the top 100 for my age classification of 50 – 54 years of age.

Will I ever do that again? Maybe not. But over my first fifty years, I've learned the dangers in saying the word "never." I still run on occasion, but now I prefer to walk, sometimes up to four and six kilometers.

Currently, I am developing a fitness program for fitness over fifty that meets all four primary needs – aerobic, resistance, flexibility and balance. Again I just need to maintain self discipline, perseverance, and patience to overcome my ego's need for me to fail. If we set aside our preconceived notions that stop us from taking action, that will help us to physically enjoy the second fifty years of our lives.

Talent without discipline is like an octopus on roller skates. There's plenty of movement, but you never know if it's going to be forward, backwards, or sideways.
H. Jackson Brown, Jr.

Setting Goals

Setting goals is the first step in turning the invisible into the visible.
Anthony Robbins

WOULD WE TAKE a two-week vacation without having any idea where we were going? Even if we had no specific destination, most of us would at least consult a map or tourist guide of the region in which we were traveling. So then why do most of us live our personal lives without any form of organized direction?

As stated earlier, it boils down to avoiding the fear and pain associated with all the effort, discipline, and time required to reach our unrealistic dreams. The reason we say "unrealistic" is because too often our dreams are based upon past or current results of another person, as well as our visual images of what they have attained. That doesn't mean these dreams aren't possible. It just means that for each of us, our starting points in all five dimensions are unique to us, and we need to be extremely careful not to overload ourselves before we have any idea of what we are getting into. That said, we still need dreams, as dreams or visions are the first step of any endeavor or plan upon which we intend to embark. However, like our vacation, our dreams need a roadmap.

We establish this roadmap by *setting goals*.

If you don't know where you are going, you'll end up someplace else.
Yogi Berra

Setting goals is the key for motivating ourselves and turning our dreams or visions into reality. The process of setting goals helps us clearly see the direction in which we need to go, how far we need to go in an allotted period of time, and keeps us focused and on course. At the same time, we are clearly defining the hazards or distractions that normally lead us down the wrong road. As well, setting and achieving goals can be incredibly motivating and an effective self-confidence builder.

A goal without a plan is just a wish.
Larry Alder

Goal setting is the ultimate high. Successful business people, world class athletes, and anyone who has achieved true success in any field, have had a well-defined plan with specific and realistically achievable goals. The process of developing and adhering to our goals gives us both long-term vision and short-term motivation. In fact setting goals helps structure our time and stay focused which ultimately helps us attain the most out of our lives.

> *Winning isn't everything, but wanting to win is.*
> **Vince Lombardi**

It's important to define our goals as clearly as possible, so we can witness our progress and accomplishments. Each personal success, no matter how small, may not have been as easily recognized had we not defined our goals. The positive feedback from accomplishing our goals also tends to steer off self-defeating behavior, that could creep in and derail the progress that we had actually already made.

> *By losing your goal, you have lost your way.*
> **Friedrich Nietzsche**

When setting our goals we should first create the big picture – that is, what we ultimately want to achieve. Now don't let this be the first stumbling block. Most of us don't have any idea of our potential, or where we really want to go. That's okay. The key is to just set a long-term goal. We can modify this goal as we discover what we are really interested in and what we want to achieve. Secondly, develop yearly, monthly, weekly and daily targets. For example, you want to attain and maintain you ideal body weight at 180 pounds, but you are currently at 204 pounds.

This is a rough guideline for weight loss goal setting, but it spells out the general idea.

Long Term Goal: To weigh and maintain 180 pounds for the rest of your life.

(To maintain 180 lbs one must eat approximately 3,500 calories per day and have a moderately active lifestyle.)

One Year Goal:	Lose 24 pounds
One Month Goal:	Lose 2 pounds per month
Weekly Goal:	Lose ½ pound a week
Daily Goal:	Reduce diet by 250 calories a day. (1,750 calories per week or ½ a pound)

(One pound of weight is equal to 3,500 calories)

When a person's goal is specifically spelled out, the task at hand doesn't seem so insurmountable. In fact, the goal becomes quite attainable, so long as we maintain honesty and self-discipline throughout the year. That doesn't mean you have to be perfect, but if you go a little overboard one day you will need to make up for it on another day. Make a mantra of these three words: *patiently, persistently* and *compassionately.*

Success is the progressive realization of a worthy goal or ideal.
Earl Nightingale

For *Your Second Fifty* lifestyle program, we will establish goals in all five dimensions:

For example,

Mental: I will learn how to program and build a website.
Emotional: I will seek to understand before being understood.
Physical: I will reduce my weight by ten pounds over the next year.
Financial: I will incorporate the money jar allocation system into my life.
Spiritual I will work daily to develop a positive outlook on life.

It's very important to try to keep goals within reach to start. To aspire to win the Tour de France in the first year of cycling may be a bit of a stretch, to say the least, but the biggest danger is that unattainable goals substantiate all the reasons why we shouldn't have even tried to do something in the first place.

The significance of a man is not in what he attains but in what he longs to attain.
Kahil Gibran

Another very important point is to make sure our goals honestly align with who we are and who we really want to be. For example, if you don't like being around children, it obviously wouldn't be advisable to return to college and study pre-school development.

If you want to be happy, set a goal that commands your thoughts, liberates your energy and inspires your hopes.
Andrew Carnegie

Review and Update Your Goals

Once we have established long-term and short-term goals, we will review and update them as needed. Keeping our ego in check here is of great importance. If we need to cut back a bit, cut back. If we need to add a bit, then add a bit. "Easy does it" and "one-step at a time" is the key to everything. Rome wasn't built in a day – nor will all these changes be easily accepted by the conscious and sub-conscious mind. But one-step at a time and easy does it will ultimately lead to attaining our goals.

Do it now. You become successful the moment you start moving toward a worthwhile goal.
Author Unknown

If we feel we are failing or not succeeding at our goals, do not worry. We simply keep moving forward. Sooner than later, we will begin to notice a shift in our behaviours and attitudes. The process and states of mind we aspired to attain will follow suit shortly thereafter.

There is one quality which one must possess to win, and that is definiteness of purpose – the knowledge of what one wants, and a burning desire to possess it.
Napoleon Hill

A few tips to consider when setting goals

When writing down your goals, *be positive*. Eliminate any negative comments or words.

Be precise, by listing dates and the amounts or values that you intend to add or reduce.

Set your goals based upon performance and not the outcome. The outcome will naturally happen if we maintain your performance levels.

Lastly, ensure that your goals line up with your true self. Determine your priorities and keep your daily goals within reach.

> *A goal properly set is halfway reached.*
> **Abraham Lincoln**

In conclusion, setting goals helps us in all areas of our lives, from determining our priorities to eliminating many distractions and irrelevant intrusions. Once we establish our first goal, our self-confidence will begin to rise. While there may be down days in the future, we will have trained ourselves that if we apply these newly acquired skills, attaining our goals is really only matter of time.

The Frank Experience - Goals

I had set goals a number of times in my life, but before 1989, I had never set *definitive* goals. Nor had I ever helped anyone else set and attain goals, until the day I sat down with my sons and planned our trip to Disneyland from our home in Victoria, British Columbia, Canada.

This trip all came about because my oldest son Scott (6 years old at the time) had been talking to a street musician at a music festival. During the conversation, he told Scott that if he and his brothers became buskers in Victoria's inner harbor, they could make as much as $100.00 a day. Now I should explain that my sons were singing on telethons and at small music festivals at the time, and they were cute and actually quite good. (My other sons are Bob, Clint and Dave – triplets - and they were 5 years old at the time.)

So Scott came to me and asked if he could sing at the harbor. I have to admit I didn't like the idea – mainly because I didn't like the fact that it might appear as if I was exploiting my sons. So I refused. About a week later, when I arrived home, there was Scott walking out the door, guitar in hand, and heading to the inner harbor. (He would have been lucky to make it there by morning if he had walked.) I told him to come back in the house and we would talk about it after dinner (hoping he would forget all about it). I was back in college at the time, and after dinner, the first book I opened was on how to be an entrepreneur. Within seconds, Scott was by my side and wanted to talk. What could I do? He wanted to be an entrepreneur. So I agreed to let him and his brothers try it out the following Saturday – but only for one hour.

During that hour they made approximately $1,000.00! The boys did nothing but talk about Disneyland all the way home on the bus. When we got home, we all sat down at the table and began the process of setting targets and goals on a big sheet of cardboard.

First we had to figure out the costs of a trip to Disneyland, renting a van (we had no car), gas, hotels, tickets, and food. After making phone calls, I determined that the cost came to approximately $6,000.00. Then we needed to add 10% to give to charity (No specific reason; just the right thing to do. We would eventually donate the money to the David Foster Foundation in Victoria). That made the total cost about $6,600.00. We then broke that number down over the 9 remaining weekends of the summer and realized that in order to make the trip, the guys would need to make $734.00 a week. To make a long story short, we left Victoria for Los Angeles the last week of August – and the boys even got to sing at Disneyland!

> *"People with goals succeed because they know where they are going. It's as simple as that."*
> **Earl Nightingale**

Mental Dimension

Rising Above the Myths of Aging – Mentally

A S WITH EVERY dimension, we will be challenged with myths and beliefs that have been passed down over time by family or friends or peers. These myths either originated to protect someone's unwillingness to put in the effort to attain success, or became convenient excuses to justify a current condition.

With today's new technology, many of these olds beliefs have been discarded... yet many people still hold on to them. Why? If we can't trust our beliefs, our entire protection system becomes questionable. And for many, that's a road they have no desire whatsoever to travel. But in order to grow, there's no choice but to move forward.

There's now a great deal of research that demonstrates when it comes to aging, your attitude makes all the difference in the world. In 2002, a Yale University study showed that women and men in their second fifty who held positive perceptions of aging lived 7.6 years longer than those who had a negative outlook.

Here are a few mental myths to be tossed under the bus.

Myth: We Lose Brain Cells as We Age

Scientists once believed that some of our brain cells died off when we got older. However, it's now clear that not only do we retain neurons, we can grow new ones, too.

Myth: Memory Loss is Inevitable as We Age

Not true. Memory loss is not an inevitable result of aging. Many doctors agree that any memory loss is likely due to some type of problem, such as a simple vitamin or hormone deficiency.

New research released at The American College of Neuropsychopharmacology's Annual Meeting found that older

Americans may improve their memory by making simple lifestyle changes – including memory exercises, physical fitness, healthy eating and stress reduction.

> *Research shows that older people tend to have lost some of their ability to pay attention, which fortunately can be improved if they work at it. The key is to - Focus, Focus, Focus!*
> **W. R. (Bill) Klemm, D.V.M., Ph.D.**

Myth: Dementia is a Normal Part of Aging

Dementia is not a normal part of aging but is caused by a number of underlying medical conditions that can occur in both elderly and younger persons.

Myth: Intelligence Declines With Age

The belief that intelligence declines with age is a flawed belief, according to the Neuroscience faculty of Macalester College. It's more a "changing of the guard" – as the dorsolateral prefrontal cortex is more active in younger adults during high cognitive load working memory tasks, whereas the rostrolateral prefrontal cortex's activity (relational integration during reasoning) actually increases in older adults.

Your Mental Dimension

> *"Intellectual growth should commence at birth and cease only at death"*
> **Albert Einstein**

Our mental dimension deals with our intellectual potential and our memory function. It's simply our ability to figure things out and retain what we have learned. Historically, the belief has been that our mental and intellectual capability deteriorates with age. However, research now shows that with proper stimulation, the brain not only maintains acceptable performance throughout its lifetime, but that it's capable of expansion and development.

In the past we were lead to believe that when brain cells died, the damage was permanent, and that the brain just deteriorated over time. However, more recent scientific research shows our brains may not only produce new brain cells or neurons throughout life, but the newly generated neurons quickly become involved in the formation of new memories.

Contrary to popular myth, you do not lose mass quantities of brains cells as you get older. "There isn't much difference between a 25-year old brain and a 75-year old brain," says Dr. Monte S. Buchsbaum, who has scanned a lot of brains as director of the Neuroscience PET Laboratory at Mount Sinai School of Medicine.

Scientific research now shows that IQ can be enhanced at any age with proper stimulation, and that our intelligence doesn't necessarily decline with age. The reason older people respond slower to questioning has more do with the fact that they are sifting through a lifetime of information than it does with diminishing mental capacities.

Scientists have now proven that the brain is plastic-like and that past views and perceptions of the brain's capabilities were somewhat off base. Michael M. Merzenich, a neuroscientist from UCSF, believes that the brain's plasticity can protect us from any physiological deterioration and overall decline in age.

The Nuns of Mankato

The brain's plasticity not only helps with recovery from injury but may actually play a role in preventing brain disease. For evidence, just visit the School Sisters of Notre Dame Nunnery in remote Mankato, Minnesota. Many are older than ninety and a surprising number reach one hundred; on average they live much longer than the general public. They also suffer far fewer, and milder, cases of Alzheimer's disease and other brain dementias. David Snowdon, the University of Kentucky professor who has been studying them for years, thinks he knows why.

Spurred on by their belief that "an idle mind is the devil's plaything," the nuns doggedly challenge themselves with vocabulary quizzes, puzzles, and debates about health care. They hold current-events seminars every week, and write often in their journals. Sister Marcella Zachman, featured in Life magazine in 1994, didn't stop teaching at the nunnery until she was ninety-seven. Sister Mary Esther Boor, also pictured in Life, still worked the front desk at ninety-nine. Snowdon, who has examined more than 100 brains donated at death by nuns in Mankato

and other School Sisters locations across the United States, maintains that the axons and dendrites that usually shrink with age branch out and make new connections if there is enough intellectual stimulation.
Excerpted from A User's Guide to the Brain: Perception, Attention, and the Four Theaters of the Brain
By John J. Ratey, M.D.

Exercise Your Brain

It's important to realize that the brain's capacity to function at a higher level is under our control. And if we want to keep our brain functioning at a higher level, we need to continually challenge ourselves with new stimulating information. As the old adage goes, "use it or lose it".

Consider your brain a muscle, and find opportunities to flex it.

"Read, read, read," says Dr. Amir Soas of Case Western Reserve University Medical School in Cleveland. "Do crossword puzzles. Play Scrabble. Start a new hobby or learn to speak a foreign language – anything that stimulates the brain to think. Also, watch less television, because your brain goes into neutral."

In the book, *Age-Proof Your Brain*, Tony Buzan indicates that the very act of learning about your brain and educating yourself about the physiology and functioning of the brain in and of itself can stimulate and compel your mind to function at a much better level.

There are countless examples of people throughout history who possessed great mental longevity. It has become a wonderful discovery that your brain has no limits in terms of its cognitive functioning, mental processing, intellect, and memory. The reality is that again you have control of all of these functions of your brain and your mind. So *if you expect your memory to deteriorate and your mental prowess to decline with age, then your expectations will be fulfilled* - this becomes a self-fulfilling prophecy.

So if you expect to gain wisdom and have incredible mental capacity throughout your life into old age, there is a high probability that this will happen to you. Remember it often takes about ten years to become an expert in something... so if you are 90 years old, you still have ten years before your Second Fifty is up, to become an expert in whatever field you choose!

It's also important to understand that the brain and body are connected, and that we can enhance our mental capacity and cognitive processing with exercise and a healthy diet. Furthermore, by improving the functioning of our brain, our emotional state will improve, which in turn will facilitate positive change throughout all the dimensions – thus improving our mood, confidence, and self-esteem.

> *Exercise increases blood flow to the brain, releases hormones, stimulates the nervous system, and increases levels of morphine like substances found in the body (such as beta-endorphin) that can have a positive effect on mood. Exercise may trigger a neurophysiological high – by giving the body a shot of adrenaline or endorphins- that produces an antidepressant effect in some, an antianxiety effect in others, and a general sense of "feeling better" in most.*
> **Michael H. Sacks, M.D.: Exercise For Stress Control**

When we discuss emotions, it's important to understand the role of the brain. Andrew Newberg, in his book *Why God Won't Go Away*, refers to the importance in differentiating between the terms "brain" and "mind." He defines the brain as a collection of physical structures that gather and process sensory, cognitive, and emotional data; whereas, the mind is the phenomenon of thoughts, memories, and emotions that arise from the perceptual processes of the brain. Without the brain's ability to process various types of input in highly sophisticated ways, the thoughts and feelings that constitute the mind would simply not exist. The brain cannot help but generate the thoughts and emotions that are the basic elements of our mind.

The mind has an incredible capacity to enter into altered states of consciousness, which may include mystical states, and the ability to interpret spiritual experiences as real. It can therefore be concluded that all that is meaningful in human spirituality happens in the mind.

Newberg states that studies show that electrical stimulation of the limbic structures in the brain produces gene-like hallucinations, out-of-body experiences and illusions, all of which occur during spiritual states. The area of the brain called the limbic system has sometimes been referred to as the "transmitter to God." The limbic system's most fundamental purpose is to generate and modulate primal emotions such as fear, aggressiveness, and rage. Other emotions like jealousy, pride, regret, embarrassment, and elation are all products of a highly developed limbic system, especially when its function is combined with the rest of the brain.

In addition, recent research shows that the mind can actually regenerate and function after brain injury. Actor and director, Christopher Reeve, known for his performances as Superman, experienced what some call a "medical marvel." On May 27, 1995, Reeve had a serious horse riding accident. The accident left him paralyzed below the neck and unable to breathe on his own. Experts predicted that Reeve would never breathe or regain the movement and feeling he had lost. In November 2000, doctor, John W. McDonald, M.D., Ph.D., watched in awe as Reeve slowly and deliberately raised the tip of his left index finger. McDonald believes that Reeve's case laid the foundation for additional studies examining the role of neural activity in regeneration and recovery of function.

The brain is an amazing organ and its functions don't need to deteriorate or decline as we age. Our brain/mind has unlimited potential regardless of age. The key is to keep exercising it, challenging it, and to change our behavior and beliefs with regard to our limitations and ability. Regardless of our age, it is important to take risks and explore new avenues.

Since 1956, the Seattle Longitudinal Study has tracked more than 5,000 people, aged 20 to 90 years old. When participants began to experience cognitive decline, they were given a series of five one-hour training sessions designed to improve inductive reasoning and spatial orientation. As a result, half of them improved cognitive functioning significantly – demonstrating that mental enrichment increases intelligence at any age.

Lead researcher of the study, Dr. K. Warner Schaie, concluded: "The results of the cognitive training studies suggest that the decline in mental performance in many community-dwelling older people is probably due to disuse and is consequently reversible."

So how do we keep our minds sharp and positive? Simple – *we exercise the brain.*

Now keep it real here. Discard the belief "if you can't be number one, there ain't no point trying." This isn't about competing with physicists or Harvard scholars – it's about living and loving life one day at a time. Challenge your mind daily. The mind is an amazing tool and the more we challenge it, the easier and more fun it becomes to address these challenges. Stick with it. Discipline is the key and you will have everything to gain. Learn a new language, read a book – fiction or non-fiction makes no difference – learn to play an instrument, or challenge the mind to question – because questioning is the key to intellectual stimulation and growth.

For growth to happen, we must remove our old ways of thinking and accept that our old beliefs may be flawed. The reality is we don't know half of what we think we know or even hope to know what we might ever know.

Your brain is the most powerful organ/instrument in your body. It has the capacity to create unbelievably wonderful experiences or moments of angst and depression. In fact your brain has the potential to completely change your whole life and your outlook on everything – instantaneously. However, you must want it – *really* want it. The more you look, the more you will find things that you enjoy.

Again Rome wasn't built in a day, nor will we develop a completely new skill overnight. But to use a cliché "we reap what we sow," and the benefits harvested will be ours to enjoy throughout our second fifty.

Your First Five Mental Footsteps

1) **Acceptance and Accountability** – So here we go, the first step! Acceptance and accountability. Do we challenge ourselves mentally? Do we read books that force us to think? Do we try to learn new things even if we have never done them before? Or are we of the mindset: "Well I did my time; I've done my part; I deserve to sit in front of a TV. I worked hard; I need to

take a rest!"

Maybe you do (or did) work hard, but sorry – that doesn't mean you should neglect or abuse your mind. If you're mentally slacking, it's time to get back in the game.

2) **Establish Goals** – So what kind of goals are we looking at here? Maybe we decide to read a new book on a subject we have no previous knowledge. Or learn to play an instrument and dedicate four hours a week to practicing? Or learn a new language? It doesn't really matter what you choose – it only matters that you choose something that will force your mind to work; something that will address new challenges and access areas of the mind that may have only had limited stimulation.

Remember, you must challenge yourself and continually increase the level of difficulty. The more you know, the more fun it becomes!

3) **Experience Your Goals** – Here the old adage applies – "use it or lose it". The mind can be compared to a muscle, in that if it is not exercised, it will shrink and become feeble.

   a. First, understand that our minds are capable of addressing anything and everything. We just need to put in the time, look at things from different perspectives, and accept that some things just take a little more time than others.
   b. Second, stay at it. Adopt the mindset, "I will get this done" and remove the all the unrealistic comparisons with others that we conjure up in our mind. The philosophy of one step at a time definitely works here.
   c. Third, accept that there is no end goal here. Continue to learn something every day of our life. Yes, you can learn something from TV, but TV watching is a passive activity – so although you are learning, your brain isn't getting any stronger. In fact, it can actually cause harm to the memory.

4) **Put Your New Skill Into Practice** – It usually takes only ten years to become an expert in something, so what the heck – become an expert at something. The interesting side to all of this is that learning become easier the more we learn. When we learn, the signals create a neural pathway through our brain. The more we learn the deeper engrained those paths become and the more efficient our mind becomes at learning. A good example would be a game trail in the bush. The more animals that use a path the more established it is and the easier it is to walk on and use.

5) **Pass It On** – Most people like to hear something new and most people respect those with factual knowledge. Once those around you begin to recognize the keenness in your eyes and the sharpness of your mind, they will become interested in how you have been able to make these adjustments. Be willing to share your experiences. Everything done has twice the value of everything read.

Remember, don't just read this book, *experience* it. In *Your Second Fifty* we only offer you direction. Try doing additional research on discipline, goals and all five dimensions. This in itself is a great way to fire up or stimulate your mental dimension.

The Frank Experience - Mental Dimension

Since turning fifty years of age, I have continually challenged my mental dimension. I became a TESOL (Teachers of English to Speakers of Other Languages) certified English teacher, a TESOL trainer, a Director of Studies at an English academy, an A&R consultant in Thailand, an Expo coordinator, learned a second language, became a communication tower installation representative, an HR Manager, a RV Salesperson, and now a trainer and an author – through all of which I had to overcome my fear of the unknown and challenge myself to experience activities in which I had limited or no previous experience. And yes at times the brain drain was intense.

But it was this book that I found most challenging. I developed the idea for *Your Second Fifty* over a three year period, but it wasn't until Michael Pond said, "Why don't you just start writing? Write a little each day and before you know it the book will be done." So off I went, compiling and structuring the data for the Fifty Fantastic Days. He was right – all it really took was to put the wheels in motion.

My original concept was to base the second fifty years around our body, mind and soul, but Mike felt the book needed a fourth dimension: emotion. We went for a drive and he helped me develop the structure of the book. I then decided to include sections on discipline and goal setting to help provide readers with the best opportunity for success. Once the structure was in place I compiled all the pertinent information and wrote my first draft. For the first three sections Mike gave me suggestions that helped establish a tone for the book. Once I had completed a section, I would pass it over to Dale for a professional read and the final structuring.

Without question I'm sure that Dale's, Mike's, and my mental dimensions were challenged just by reading what I had written. However, in order to complete this book I needed to apply self-discipline and to set challenging but attainable goals as well. The puzzle could not have been completed without applying all of the pieces.

The book was originally released in S.E. Asia in 2009 and was a best seller. When my father and mother became ill, I returned to Canada to assist them. While here in Canada, I came to the conclusion that one more dimension was required to make *Your Second Fifty* complete – Financial. I believe that without financial peace of mind, people will never be free to fully engage and grow in the other four dimensions. So, I added the Financial Dimension.

I firmly believe that so long as I continue to challenge myself to overcome my fears, I will continue to expand my mental dimension, throughout the second fifty years of my life.

The power of thought, the magic of the mind.
Byron Lord

Emotional Dimension

Rising Above the Myths of Aging - Emotionally

PERSONALLY I STRUGGLED with my emotional dimension until I started to write *Your Second Fifty*. And yes, some days I still do! That said, I'm now fully aware that if it's to be – it's up to me! My emotions are created by myself and acted upon because of my choice. And that wasn't an easy pill to swallow at first.

Here are a few emotional myths that need to be tossed in the trash can.

Myth: Expressing an Emotion Will Get Rid of It.

This myth is unfortunately touted by many mental health professionals. Sure it may feel at the moment that you've released it, however it will return as soon as the same scenario or beliefs that sparked it in the first place return. The only real way to make lasting change is if a person changes their perception and interpretation of the situation that triggered the emotion in the first place. Same problem, same solution, same result, same pain!

Myth: Emotions Are Irrational.

Emotions arise from our beliefs, which are related to past experiences and are directly related to our thinking. The only way an emotion becomes irrational is when we have based them on faulty reasoning or our inaccurate perceptions. An emotion is more apt to be rational and appropriate when they are based upon accurate reasoning and holistic views.

Myth: Either We Control or Indulge Our Emotions.

Attempting to exert too much control of our emotions can lead to unhappiness and depression. Indulging our emotions can lead to internal frustration and despair. Simply accepting an emotion for what it is would mean that every emotion is true and valid – and that's simply not the case. The healthy approach is to manage our emotions, to understand them through the process of introspection, and then decide if and how we want to choose to respond to them.

Myth: Other People Affect Our Emotions.

Many people believe that their emotions are triggered by what happens outside of them, such as situations and events – or far too often, the actions of other people. But, the truth is that it's not other people's behaviors or actions that make us feel something. *It's how we think about their other person's actions.* Once we understand and accept that other people don't control our emotions, we actually regain control over our lives. From there we can decide how and if we want to address and react to the situation.

Your Emotional Dimension

> *"...in navigating our lives, it is our fears and envies, our rages and depressions, our worries and anxieties that steer us day to day. Even the most academically brilliant among us are vulnerable to being undone by unruly emotions. The price we pay for emotional literacy is in failed marriages and troubled families, in stunted social and work lives, in deteriorating physical health and mental anguish..."*
> **Daniel Goleman**

The world has become an increasingly difficult place to live. If we haven't the skills to maintain proper control over our emotions, our lives will spiral out of control and we will be stuck in the rut of casting blame either inward or outward.

> *The evidence has been piling up throughout history, and now neuroscientists have proved it's true: the brain's wiring emphatically relies on emotion over intellect in decision-making.*
> **http://www.usatoday.com/tech/science/discoveries/2006-08-06-brain-study_x.htm**

Most people believe that emotions are caused by events and outside sources. They are in fact caused by our *perceptions and interpretations of events* – sometimes so fleeting and fast as to be beneath the level of consciousness. Our pre-conscious, split-second thoughts give rise to automatic emotional reactions to which we may or may not have already attached a specific response. We then have a choice as to how we behave, what we say, and how we handle a situation. The appropriateness of our actions and the effectiveness of our communications make up our emotional intelligence.

People who are highly developed emotionally become sensitive to pre-conscious thoughts, question their validity and appropriateness, and are able to directly influence their feelings, personal beliefs and behaviors. People who are less developed are at times slaves to their emotions.

> *"Our beliefs create the world that we live in, and our beliefs and thoughts therefore also create the stress we experience. If we think something is safe and possible to conquer, then it is. But if we think the opposite then that will be our experiences."*
> **Janice Calnan, Psychotherapist**

Western culture has adopted the philosophy that it's all or nothing. 2nd place is unacceptable and can only be perceived as the 1st place loser. This unrealistic belief and expectation ultimately leads to criticism somewhere down the road and its fear of this criticism that leads to stress. Understand is that stress can be addictive, and that this stress can have a direct result on the aging of our body and mind.

Also understand that the event or situation that we believe caused the stress is not really the cause of the stress. Stress is created by our own mental and emotional experience of the event or situation. This means you create your own stress. The good news is that with proper management of our emotions, we can reduce stress, which in turn reduces the additional wear and tear on our minds and bodies. Also, researchers have concluded that people who deal effectively with others and exercise proper control over their own emotions are more likely to live happy lives.

What to Improve Our Emotional Control

To start it would be a good idea to take an EQ (Emotional Quotient) test to understand your strengths and vulnerabilities. These tests are readily available on the Internet for a cost; however, if you purchase *The Emotional Intelligence Quick Book* by Travis Bradberry and Jean Greaves – an online EQ test is included with in the purchase price of the book.

> **Emotional Intelligence (EI)** = *Understanding and Managing your Feelings and Emotions*
> **Emotional Quotient (EQ)** = *Like IQ, a measure of one's emotional knowledge and understanding.*

Within the discussion of Emotional Intelligence there are many definitions and terms. However, for our purpose we will utilize the following as defined by Daniel Goleman:

> **Self-awareness** - the ability to read one's emotions and recognize their impact while using gut feelings to guide decisions.
> **Self-management** - involves controlling one's emotions and impulses and adapting to changing circumstances.
> **Social awareness** - the ability to sense, understand, and react to other's emotions while comprehending social networks.
> **Relationship management** - the ability to inspire, influence, and develop others while managing conflict.

Once we have an understanding of our strengths and vulnerabilities, we will learn to identify the causes of our feelings and to become aware of our preconscious thoughts. Emotions are automatic responses to previously determined value judgments – therefore, if we carefully evaluate how we explained this situation to ourselves in the past, we can proactively prepare for the next time this emotion arises.

Here are a couple of examples: If we didn't have a belief that traffic should move quickly, then we wouldn't get angry when traffic slowed down. Traffic simply is what it is. It is our preconceived view of "how the traffic is supposed to move" that upsets us, not the traffic itself. Similarly, nobody makes us angry. We make ourselves angry by expecting people to act the way we want them to act and then us not accepting them the way they are.

The more aware we become of our emotions and associated reactions the better equipped we become at stemming and preventing situations that we may regret at some point later on in the future.

Valerie Cox's poem "The Cookie Thief" puts a unique twist on the dangers of impulsive emotional reactions.

The Cookie Thief

A woman was waiting at an airport one night,
With several long hours before her flight.
She hunted for a book in the airport shops.
Bought a bag of cookies and found a place to drop.

She was engrossed in her book but happened to see,
That the man sitting beside her, as bold as could be.
Grabbed a cookie or two from the bag in between,
Which she tried to ignore to avoid a scene.

So she munched the cookies and watched the clock,
As the gutsy cookie thief diminished her stock.
She was getting more irritated as the minutes ticked by,
Thinking, "If I wasn't so nice, I would blacken his eye."

With each cookie she took, he took one too,
When only one was left, she wondered what he would do.
With a smile on his face, and a nervous laugh,
He took the last cookie and broke it in half.

He offered her half, as he ate the other,
She snatched it from him and thought... oooh, brother.
This guy has some nerve and he's also rude,
Why he didn't even show any gratitude!

She had never known when she had been so galled,
And sighed with relief when her flight was called.
She gathered her belongings and headed to the gate,
Refusing to look back at the thieving ingrate.

She boarded the plane, and sank in her seat,
Then she sought her book, which was almost complete.
As she reached in her baggage, she gasped with surprise,
There was her bag of cookies, in front of her eyes.

If mine are here, she moaned in despair,
The others were his, and he tried to share.
Too late to apologize, she realized with grief,
That she was the rude one, the ingrate, the thief.
Valerie Cox

Trust your natural instincts to understand what emotion it is that is arising at any given moment and be prepared to provide a positive response. Better yet, simply observe the emotion until it dissipates and passes.

The key to observing emotions as they arise is to understand and accept that emotions can appear quickly and intensely. The emotion itself is only a sensation; it's we who insist on labeling it and giving it direction and a life of its own. Once we master the skill of observation, we will notice that when we become aware of the sensation rising, we don't need to react or respond because that sensation will fade just as quickly as it came.

How Does Exercise Affect Emotion?

In a recent study researchers have found that physical activity provides significant emotional benefits to people with personalities that tend to be more negative, anxious and depressed. Peter Giacobbi Jr., an assistant professor of sport and exercise psychology at the University of Florida's College of Health and Human Performance said, "We found that regardless of the events they experienced on any given day, they had an increased positive mood and a decreased negative mood on a day they exercised more. And that was pretty powerful."

Again, developing and balancing our five dimensions will lead us to a happy and healthier lifestyle.

James Blumenthal and a team of researchers at Duke University Medical Center found that an aerobic exercise program decreased depression and improved the cognitive abilities of middle-aged and elderly men and women. They followed 156 patients between the ages of 50 and 77 who had been diagnosed with major depressive disorder. They were randomly assigned to one of three groups: exercise, medication, or a combination of medication and exercise. The exercise group spent 30 minutes either riding a stationary bicycle or walking, or jogging three times a week. To the surprise of the researchers, after 16 weeks, all three groups showed statistically significant and identical improvement in standard measurements of depression.

Story of the Two Monks

Two monks were making a pilgrimage. During the course of their journey, they came to a river where they met a beautiful young woman – an apparently worldly creature, dressed in expensive finery and with her hair done up in the latest fashion. She was afraid of the current and afraid of ruining her lovely clothing, so asked the brothers if they might carry her across the river.

The younger and more exacting of the brothers was offended at the very idea and turned away with an attitude of disgust. The older brother didn't hesitate, and quickly picked the woman up on his shoulders, carried her across the river, and set her down on the other side. She thanked him and went on her way, and the brother waded back through the waters.

The monks resumed their walk, the older one in perfect equanimity and enjoying the beautiful countryside, while the younger one grew more and more brooding and distracted, so much so that he could keep his silence no longer and suddenly burst out, "Brother, we are taught to avoid contact with women, and there you were, not just touching a woman, but carrying her on your shoulders!"

The older monk looked at the younger with a loving smile and said, "Brother, I set her down on the other side of the river; you are still carrying her."

Your First Five Emotional Footsteps

1) **Acceptance and Accountability** – This is the hardest step we will take in personal self-growth. In this step we must be as honest as we possibly can be so that the path we lay out will lead us to where we really want to go. Here we need look in

the mirror and ask: "Do I have the courage to honestly begin to look at my strengths and vulnerabilities and am I ready and willing to begin this journey? Just how much control do I have over my emotions? Do I have occasional outbursts or do I maintain calmness in the face of adversity?"

Today more than ever we need to realize that getting things off our chest via emotional outbursts of any sort, won't accomplish what we've been lead to believe in the past. Venting our frustrations on others doesn't make us feel better; in fact, it usually makes us feel worse.

A perfect example is getting cut off in traffic. We curse, display obscene gestures, and loathe the person – possibly for hours. And does this make us feel better? Absolutely not. In fact, all we've done is add additional stress and wear and tear to our bodies from our inability to control our emotions.

The key is to effectively communicate to others how we feel – what emotions we are experiencing and then ask them to refrain from acting in a way that we perceive as harmful.

When we learn to properly control our emotions, we enhance our compassion. And with greater compassion, we are capable of considering possible alternatives as to why the person acted in the manner that they did. Once we consider these options we reduce the self-serving anger that is associated in perceiving that the whole situation was in fact an act against us.

2) **Establish Goals** – Come to a clear understanding as to what are our strengths and vulnerabilities. This is best understood after completing an EQ test. Look around and choose a test that we are comfortable in doing. Not only will this search give us a diversified perspective and more complete knowledge of EQ, but the process of searching will also be a positive stimulus for your mental dimension. Once you have completed the test you can then determine what areas of your EI (Emotional Intelligence) you want to focus on and improve. If you are still unsure, consult friends and family for ideas.

3) **Experience Your Goals** – There is no short cut or quick fix. Experience your goals one step at a time. Apply self-discipline.

    a. First, observe the sensations that are happening in your body just prior to our emotional responses and reactions. Be patient as this will take time, if you are feeling impatient with your progress, observe those sensations.

    b. Second, observe the emotional responses and reactions that follow these sensations. Again this may take time, but soon enough patterns will begin to emerge.

    c. Third, question yourself to try and understand where and when it was in your life that you established your responses and reactions to specific sensations. For example: You dislike your brother's friend with the red hair, and when he came over, you always wanted to leave the house. Now as you are older, when you see a person with red hair, you have a strange sensation and then you feel the urge to leave.

    d. Fourth, be willing to question yourself to see if your reaction is valid, or if you established and based your response upon false or inaccurate information. Obviously, not all people with red hair pose a threat or warrant running from.

    e. Fifth, decide if the reaction is of a benefit to you or not. If your reaction isn't going to provide you with a positive result, it's best to just continue to observe it and let it dissolve and disappear. All emotions come and go relatively quickly, it's our beliefs, behavior and actions that give them life, validity, and reality.

4) **Putting Our New Skill Into Practice** – The good news is that once we realize we have the ability to control our emotions; life begins to become more manageable. Our fight or flight behavior* begins to subside and our acceptance of ourselves and others begins to increase. Self-destructive behavior will of course attempt to re-establish itself; however, our new skills in addition to our goals and self-discipline will diminish the effect negative emotional reactions have over us. As we continue to question the validity of our responses, our compassion will begin to increase as we consider the other person's point of view. With increased compassion, comes peace of heart and greater happiness. A great meditation style for learning how to observe and deal with sensations and following emotions is Vipassana Meditation.

* *The fight-or-flight response, also called hyperarousal or the acute stress response, was first described by Walter Cannon in 1915. His theory states that animals react to threats with a general discharge of the sympathetic nervous system, priming the animal for fighting or fleeing.* **http://en.wikipedia.org/wiki/Fight_or_flight**

Pass It On – *Your Second Fifty* consists of simple, but long term lifestyle shifts. With today's society geared for the quick fix, those of us willing to take up the challenge may appear to be walking a long and lonely path. However, once we begin to observe our emotional behaviour shift, the laws of natural attraction will soon begin to take place. Other people's opinions will take on a new light and we will be interested in hearing them. Our need to be right will diminish, making us more appealing to others.

The key to our emotional growth is our awareness. We must remain aware of our emotions if we hope to control them, and once we do others will certainly be attracted to our new found happiness. Remember the old cliché "you can take a horse to water, but you can't make it drink," or "when the student is ready the teacher will appear". The key is to tell everyone about the possibilities that lie before them and then let them decide for themselves. All we need to do is lead by example, and they will be certain to try sooner or later. Attract rather than promote!

Happiness is never obtained from succeeding to be right – this is one of life's greatest illusions.
Frank Moffatt

The Frank Experience – Emotional Dimension

In my past, I was always willing to argue or fight. I was aggressive, domineering and always needed to be right. Now I can say that while those emotions still do arise from time to time, I can usually see them coming – and prior to reacting, disengage them. That doesn't mean I allow others to inflict their negativity or frustrations upon me – because I don't – but now I try to deal from the truth and not my ego. Today I have a choice: I can either provide a positive resolve, or walk away, because I do know that conflict resolves nothing.

In 2004, I went on my first ten-day silent meditational retreat and learned a great deal about my emotions. What I learned served me well for a couple of years, but without self-discipline and a support system to maintain consistent practice, I ended up slipping and falling back towards some of my old behavioral patterns. It took a while to get back on track, and a second course, but again I'm practicing and applying emotional awareness and control to my daily life. It was easier this time because of my previously established patterns and understanding.

By no means am I a perfect person. However, each day that I attempt to maintain awareness of my emotions and work at enhancing my emotional intelligence, I have a much greater chance of not offending others. And so long as I don't accept another person's frustration, anger, or hate, what possible chance do they have of offending me?

Well, I don't accept your insult, so it returns to you.
Buddha

Physical Dimension

Rising Above the Myths of Aging - Physically

OVER THE PAST year I helped my father lose 55 pounds. He could only walk 6 steps before needing a rest, complained of leg pain daily, was a candidate for oxygen and his doctors weren't giving him much more than a few months to live. Today he has very little leg pain, doesn't require oxygen, can walk around the entire mall unassisted and his doctors are amazed with the change in his health. Although he did have a coach (me) and he likely wouldn't have made these changes himself, that's not the point. The point is that by changing his physical condition, his life has improved and many of his ailments are no longer an issue.

Here are a few physical myths that need to be tossed in the trash can.

Myth: Creaky, Achy Joints are Unavoidable

The real truth about aching bones is a lack of exercise. Australian researchers at the Monash University Medical School found that women ages 40 to 67 that exercised at least once every two weeks for 20 minutes had more cartilage in their knees – suggesting that being physically active in your second fifty made it less likely that you would develop arthritis.

Myth: We Lose Our Desire for Sex as We Age

Impotence and reduced libido are not so much age-related as they are responses to preventable medical conditions like depression, diabetes, high blood pressure and heart disease. The key to a healthy sex life is keeping your body healthy and fit. In fact, something as simple as walking daily and lifting weights a two or three times a week can dramatically improve your sexual desire. That said, sexual desire might decline a little once you hit 75, however according to a report by the New Jersey Institute for Successful Aging, addressing mature adults over 60 years of age, 60 percent had regular physical and sexual experiences in the past year. And they all wanted more!

Myth: Your Bones Become Fragile and Your Posture Bends

Only death is certain when it comes to aging. Osteoporosis is more common in older people, but it is preventable. Studies have shown that just over 50% of females over 100 years of age had osteoporosis, and that their average age of diagnosis was 87. Keep in mind these women knew little about the benefits of diet and exercise and how they affected their bones.

Myth: Women Lose Their Ability to Achieve an Orgasm in Their Second Fifty

Statistics show that the "Golden Age" for women hovers between 65 to 75 years of age. In fact, sex in their second fifty can become more emotionally and physically satisfying than ever before.

Myth: Your Families Genes Determine How You'll Age

Sorry this just isn't true. Regardless of the health of your genes, how you live your life will determine your lifespan. Genes can be changed by your diet, physical activity and even your exposure to chemicals.

Myth: Men Lose Their Ability to Achieve an Erection in Their Second Fifty

Despite diminishing hormone levels, older men remain entirely capable of having healthy, active sex lives. And now with options like Cialis and Viagra there's no need to ever stop.

Your Physical Dimension

It has been scientifically proven that there is nothing in the body that causes it to age. There are no time-released elements, or alarm clocks set to go off at specific times causing deterioration. The reason people age in appearance and attitude is because they believe they're supposed to. They've programmed themselves subconsciously to look and act a certain way at respective points in their lives. They believe and accept age and therefore get old.
Jean Walters

Do you accept Jean Walter's comment? Do you have the courage to look outside of the box and admit that what you have come to believe may indeed not be the truth? In fact do you have the willingness to consider that the way you feel today may not even be the tip of your unlimited physical potential?

In the book "BioMarkers" by William Evans, Harvard Medical School has proved that the body completely rebuilds itself and can actually grow younger. So how long does it take your body to replace every cell in it? <u>Seven years</u>. In Deepak Chopra's book, *Quantum Healing*, he states that our liver completely rebuilds itself every 6 weeks; our skeleton every 3 months; our stomach lining every 4 days and our skin every month.

Physical fitness is not only finely interwoven with your intellectual, emotional, financial and spiritual dimensions, but plays an important role in maintaining overall well-being.

A major five-year study at the Laval University in Sainte-Foy, Quebec, of 5,000 men and women over age 65, demonstrated that those who exercise regularly are less likely to show a decline in mental performance. Those who did not exercise and lived a more sedentary lifestyle were more likely to experience mental degenerative disorders.

> *The word exercise derives from a Latin root meaning "to maintain, to keep, to ward off." To exercise means to practice, put into action, train, perform, use, and improve.*

In this section we will explore the physical dimension and the choices of healthy activities and alternatives that lay before us when considering our own person fitness programs.

We suggest that a fitness program provides a sensible balance between feeling good when one looks in the mirror and feeling good after one has participated in some form of exercise or activity. Keep in mind that physically fit bodies take time to develop. If we focus on the end result of our goal the task will appear insurmountable, but if we go about it one day at a time, before one knows it we will have enough improvement to have a new appreciation for our physical self. Take it easy – have fun.

Here are a few tips to consider when exercising:

- Exercise for YOU! Don't subject yourself to self-professing experts. Everyone has an opinion, and while his or her intent may be honorable, spare yourself from his or her kindness. If you really need help to develop a program seek out a professional trainer at your local gym or from the internet directory. At the end of this section we will provide you with a number of options that will hopefully assist you in your search for expanded awareness and understanding of your Physical Dimension.

- Go about things slowly and trust your body to let you know what is right and what is not right for you. How will you know if what you are doing is right? Trust yourself, follow the instructions for whatever exercise you have chosen (a number of exercises are listed near the back of this book) and take it easy.

- Listen to your body, it will tell you if the movement feels acceptable and if the weight or resistance is safe. Again if you're not comfortable, seek out a professional until you have developed enough confidence to trust yourself. In any case, only you will know if you are being honest with yourself. Once that honesty has been developed, self-trust will soon follow.

The National Institute on Aging states that osteoporosis is a preventable disorder when weight-bearing exercises such as "walking, jogging, playing tennis and dancing," become lifestyle activities done three to four times per week.

Keep active! Working out and cardiovascular exercise are non-negotiable options when it comes to improving and maintaining physical health. Resistance training (weight training) needs to be based on an ever increasing resistance program, so the body will have an opportunity to maintain or even gain bone density and muscle mass. That being said, one needs to be patient and increase resistance slowly.

Nothing puts a bigger dent into the start of a new workout program than an injury, and all the self-defeating behavior that accompanies it.

Aging Well, NY State

Not long ago, it was "accepted knowledge" that older people could not increase their muscle strength nor their muscle mass. Now, happily, this myth has been dispelled. In 1989, researchers from Tufts and Harvard Universities undertook a study of older people in their late 80's and 90's. They did three sets composed of eight weight lifting repetitions each for three days a week.

After two weeks, they were retested and the weights were increased. At the end of six weeks, these frail older people had increased their muscle strength on average by 180 percent. What is more interesting, none of the participants had reached a plateau. As a result of their increased muscle strength, their average walking speed increased 48 percent. Two participants no longer needed their canes, and one participant was able to rise from a chair without using the chair arms.

All of the participants resumed their sedentary lifestyles at the end of the program. The researchers then retested them, and found a 32 percent loss in maximum strength after only 4 weeks without training. The moral of this story is "If you don't use it, you'll lose it." But the happy ending is that you can regain your fitness and strength at almost any age which will help you to retain or regain your independence, freedom, and add to your good looks.

Adapted From: "Fitness Facts for Older Americans,"
Source: New York State Office for the Aging, 1998

Balance and stretching exercises also play a key role in maintaining the physical component of our lives. A great way to accomplish both goals would be to attend yoga or Tai Chi classes a couple of times a week. Again remember, Rome wasn't built in a day. Go about your program one day at a time. Before you know it you'll be pleasantly surprised with your newly acquired flexibility, balance and strength.

An additional benefit to improved overall balance is the reduced fear of falling.

"People have the mistaken idea that exercise is a fabulous way to lose weight," says William Evans of the University of Arkansas for Medical

Sciences. "But exercising doesn't burn a lot of calories." Walking or running a mile burns about 100 calories. But sitting still for the same time burns about 50 or 60 calories. "So the extra you expend isn't huge and people get discouraged at their slow rate of weight loss."

You don't need a day off

I repeat: you don't need a day off. Stay active and live life to the fullest. The only people that benefit from a sedentary society are furniture salesmen and convenience stores. You gain nothing from being a couch potato. You don't deserve any of the self-inflicted diseases, aches and pains associated with lethargic behavior. Keep this in mind: as human beings we are innately lazy. That's just the way it is. Therefore, we must take the initiative to make things happen. We will never be free in life until we take full responsibility and ownership of our lives.

So the first step in taking responsibility is to build ourselves a weekly workout routine.

Workout   **Routine**   **Example**
(Expanded Examples are located in Appendex A)

Monday	Aerobics	Brisk walk or yoga
Tuesday	Resistance Training	Chest, back & shoulders
Wednesday	Aerobics	Water aerobics
Thursday	Resistance Training	Legs, arms and abdominal
Friday	Aerobics	Tennis, Badminton or yoga
Saturday	Resistance Training	Chest, back & shoulders
Sunday	A walk in the park, gardening, or mall shopping	

Following Week (Switch things up a bit):

Monday	Resistance Training	Chest, back & shoulders
Wednesday	Resistance Training	Legs, arms and abdominal
Friday	Resistance Training	Chest, back & shoulders
Tuesday	Resistance Training	Legs, arms and abdominal
Thursday	Resistance Training	Chest, back & shoulders
Saturday	Resistance Training	Legs, arms and abdominal

Add stretching and balance exercises daily at the end of your workout.

Whatever program you choose to use for yourself will be the right program, so long as you take it easy to start and pay attention to your body and what it is telling you. As you gain experience with exercising, you will make adjustments based upon observations you make about your body. There is no right and wrong in choosing exercises so long as you follow the proper steps for each exercise. Just remember, it is always healthier to do *something* than to do nothing at all!

Establish a Healthy, Well-balanced Diet

The first thing to understand is what your body needs nutritionally. The key to achieving and maintaining nutritional health is to know what, when, and how much to eat.

Choices should be:

- ❖ Of moderate calorie content, nutrient-dense: low in fat and sodium and high in fiber and calcium.
- ❖ Tasty so you enjoy them.
- ❖ Easy to chew, swallow, and digest.
- ❖ Easy to make.
- ❖ Pleasing to look at.

Stay away from processed foods and stick to natural food products.

- ❖ Focus on good carbohydrates. Choose whole grain (brown rice, whole wheat bread, rolled oats, barley, millet). Stay away from "white" products, such as white rice, white bread and products made with white flour and white sugar.

- ❖ Eat raw fruits and vegetables. Try to eat at least two daily serving of raw fruits and vegetables, as they contain the highest nutritional value. If you wish to cook your vegetables steaming is best as it doesn't cook out the nutrients.

- ❖ Keep the protein lean. Fish, poultry, eggs, beans, peas, nuts, and seeds are all healthy sources of protein. Bake, broil, grill, steam, or poach your meal to help you maintain a healthy, low-fat, low cholesterol diet. Yes – frying is <u>out</u>!

❖ Consume calcium from natural sources. Milk, cheese, and yogurt are all excellent sources of calcium, whereas cream cheese, cream, and butter are not. If possible purchase fat-free or low fat dairy products and limit the amount you eat to what is acceptable.

❖ Choose healthy fats. Olive oil and sunflower oil, avocados and avocado oil, nuts and seeds are all great.

❖ Hydrating your body. A suitable allowance of **water** for adults is 2.5 litres **daily** in most instances. In addition to drinking water, consumption of high water content foods such as melons, grapes, cucumbers, onions and apples help to keep us properly hydrated and flush toxins from the body, while keeping our joints flexible and our minds clear.

"Where is the beef and where is the bacon?"

Well again that's up to you. Moderation is the key to healthy living. No one is saying you shouldn't have a piece of chocolate cake at your son's birthday or a nice thick juicy steak at the family reunion. A calorie is a calorie so indulging every now and then certainly isn't worth the grief or guilt many of us have grown accustom to heaping on ourselves when we slip up a bit. In fact it has been proven if you don't indulge every now and then you ego will certainly sabotage your best efforts.

The key is actually to become aware of what, when, and where we are eating at all times. Too often we find ourselves eating, not because we are hungry, but because we are trying to suppress another emotion that is stirring inside. Food fuels our body like gasoline fuels our car, put in the wrong grade and your car will ping as you drive down the road. So think about it, you can either ping or purr through life and that choice is 100% up to you.

Calories in One Pound of Body Weight

It takes about 3,500 calories to make 1 pound. This pertains to whether they are food calories coming in, or calories (burned by exercise) going out. If you eat 3,500 calories more than your body needs, you will gain about 1 pound. If you use up 3,500 calories more than you eat, you will lose about 1 pound.

Calories Needed Per Day

Here is a simple formula to use as an estimate for your daily calorie requirements:

- ❖ Change your weight from pounds to kilograms: Divide total pounds by 2.2
- ❖ The average person's basal metabolic rate is approximately 1 calorie per kilogram per hour. Multiply your weight in kilograms by the 24 hours in a day. You will burn this many calories just staying alive.
- ❖ Now factor in your additional daily calorie consumption based upon your activity level:

Light activity: 50% to 70%
Moderate: 65% to 80%
Heavy: 90% to 120%

- ❖ If you have a desk job and workout 30 minutes per day, this would be considered light activity. Most North Americans fit into this class.
- ❖ If your job involves physical activity and you are physically active in addition to your workout (walk to work, use the stairs, etc.), this would be moderate.
- ❖ Construction workers, athletes, etc. would be considered heavy activity.
- ❖ Once you have calculated your basic calories needed to stay alive, add them to your activity calories and you will have an approximation as to the number of calories you need per day.

Example:

If you weigh 180 pounds, divide by 2.2 to get 81.81 kilograms (round up or down if you wish).

> 81.81 x 24 hours = **1963.63** calories needed per day for basic function.

Let's say you're activity is <u>light</u>.

> 1963.63 plus 50% = 2945.44 (2945)
> 1963.63 plus 70% = 3338.17 (3338)

So for a person weighing 180 pounds that is lightly active, they would burn between 2945 to 3338 calories per day. To lose weight, you need to burn more calories than you eat, by either eating less or exercising more.

One Potentially Dangerous Fast Food Day:

Breakfast

Bran Muffin 5oz:	405
Orange Juice 1 cup:	100

Lunch

Hamburger:	500
French Fries:	500
Coca Cola – 12oz/ 375 ml can:	200

Dinner

Large Taco:	500
Tortilla chips, taco, 8oz:	1,100
Cookies & Cream (Haagen-Dazs) ½ cup:	270

Evening

Beer (3):	315
Pretzels, 8oz:	900

Total Calorie Intake: 4,790

This would equal nearly a 1/2 of a pound gain for a 180-pound man, whose daily activity was light.

A reasonable indicator for your healthy weight range is the Body Mass Index (BMI). The BMI is a measure of body fat based on height and weight that applies to both adult men and women. You can find BMI tables on the internet.

For those of you that consider yourself big boned, sorry but there is no scientific data to substantiate that big bones have any significant effect on one's overall weight classification or BMI. Just another one of those myths…

Identifying and Eliminating Mental Road Blocks

Everything that we do in our lives is linked mentally, emotionally, physically, financially and spiritually. So even if we were to follow the greatest workout program ever designed and strictly follow the ultimate diet, our physical gains may still fall short of our expectations if we don't have a positive physical image of ourselves. And why might that be you ask? Perhaps it's that we don't sub-consciously believe we are worth it.

It's a scientifically-proven fact that our subconscious mind doesn't know the difference between what's real and what's imagined. So the good news is that we have the ability to change our self-image and our external image to anything we want, provided it falls in line with who we really are and our core beliefs of who we really want to be.

In fact, anything we focus our thoughts on the mind will start the process of creating it. That is unless we have a stronger negative view from our emotional self that overrides this process. That negativity could be based upon a fear attached to our projected image; it could be that our image is not in agreement with whom we really are; it could be based on the values of others; or the guilt based "I should". If there is any conflict between your desired self and your internal self-image, your goals may be quite difficult to attain… BUT not impossible!

Positive self-imaging that is in line with who we really are has the potential to erase this conflict. Remember, negative thoughts lead to negative results and positive thoughts lead to the positive possibility of change and a newly enhanced self-image. So who are you? A **Good Person**!

Self-imaging is developed by the mind, ignited by emotions, incorporated into the body, facilitated through finances and inspired by faith. Once we have consciously and subconsciously developed the image of who we want to be, we add the other elements to bring our image into a five dimensional reality. Hence, we become our image. This does work, so long as we are completely honest with our self.

Once we've reached this level of actualization, we must maintain our new self-image, by confronting and resolving any beliefs, behaviors or patterns that challenge our new image of ourselves. Certainly there will be challenges and disillusionment along the way, as there is in any endeavor. However, be assured these are only momentary setbacks and you will bounce back on track and in line with your newly acquired self-image. Things sometimes look bad before turning the corner to reward and success. It's those that persevere that reap the rewards Those that quit or procrastinate, don't.

Stress

With an improved self-image, comes an enhanced awareness of how to deal with life's daily challenges and stresses. However until that awareness of your new self-image is firmly entrenched, be aware of the effects of stress on weight control and management. When we are stressed we can gain weight even if we haven't increased the amount of food we are consuming. Stress produces cortisol, which slows metabolism, resulting in a weight gain.

When we experience chronic stress we tend to crave more fatty, salty, and sugary foods, which include sweets and processed foods. The fat we store when stressed tends to be stored as abdominal fat, which presents greater health risks than fat stored on the other parts of our body.

Alternative Fitness Options

Fitness comes in many forms and not only from lifting weights, running, swimming and riding a bike. Keep your eyes and ears open. Be willing to try and experience something new.

Massage

There are a numerous massage therapy techniques available to gently nurture your body.

- ❖ **Swedish Massage** – utilizes tapping and kneading strokes to work the entire body to relieve muscle tension and loosen sore joints.

- ❖ **Thai massage** – utilizes various stretches and acupressure points to increase flexibility, release muscle tension and energy blocks.

- ❖ **Deep Tissue Massage** – utilizes slow strokes and direct pressure or friction movements that go across the grain of the muscles to relieve chronic tension.

- ❖ **Rolfing** - utilizes hands and elbows to realign and straighten the body by working the myofascia, the connective tissue surrounding your muscles and holding your body together.

An increasing number of research studies show massage reduces heart rate, lowers blood pressure, increases blood circulation and lymph flow, relaxes muscles, improves range of motion, and increases endorphins (enhancing medical treatment). Although therapeutic massage does not increase muscle strength, it can stimulate weak, inactive muscles and, thus, partially compensate for the lack of exercise and inactivity resulting from illness or injury. It also can hasten and lead to a more complete recovery from exercise or injury.
www.holisticonline.com

Yoga

Yoga has long been accepted as an excellent way to enhance one's mental, emotional, physical and spiritual dimensions. We highly recommend that you consider joining a yoga class.

There are many different types of yoga, each with their own focus and benefits. For more information, visit a local yoga studio, or do some research online. One good website for information on yoga is YogaUOnline.com.

Yoga, an ancient but perfect science, deals with the evolution of humanity. This evolution includes all aspects of one's being, from bodily health to self-realization. Yoga means union - the union of body with consciousness and consciousness with the soul. Yoga cultivates the ways of maintaining a balanced attitude in day-to-day life and endows skill in the performance of one's actions.
~**B.K.S. Iyengar, Astadala Yogamala**

Your First Five Physical Footsteps

1) **Acceptance and Accountability** – Your first physical step should be either step on to a scale, or in front of a full size mirror, <u>naked</u>. Are we happy? Certainly not if we are comparing ourselves with all the airbrushed models on today's magazines. So, it's time to get realistic. There's no need to be a sex goddess, just be healthy. If we are fat, we are fat. If we eat unhealthy foods, we are unhealthy. It is what it is. If we are overweight and unhealthy, accept it and shed all the excuses as to why we are the way we are. Accept and be accountable.

2) **Establish Goals** – What is it we really want? Are our everyday tasks a burden? Do we have aches and pains that we would love to be rid of? Do we feel sluggish and uninspired? All of these hassles and pains can be greatly reduced by exercise. So let's get started. We need a balanced program to include cardio, strength and stretching & balance exercises. One hour a day five days a week is plenty. In fact a 20-20-20 minute program is ideal to start.

To build your program, look at the exercises at the back of the book and try and do one exercise per body part per workout. Remember this is fitness training for overall health – not competitive training for bodybuilding or to run in a marathon. It would be a good idea to write down your specific goals, whatever they may be. Take it easy to start, we don't want to give ourselves an excuse to quit right off of the top. If you've had health issues in the past or are unsure about your health, it would be wise to consult a doctor prior to exercising.

3) **Experience Your Goals** – You can read all you want about fitness, eat all the supplements in the world, but if you don't live the experience there is no possible way to reap the rewards.

    a. First, organize the exercises you have chosen for that day onto a list. Leave room so you can add the weights you chose in the next step. This will help keep things flowing smooth each time you train. Do Cardio first, strength second, and stretching & balance third.

    b. Second, test the weights to ensure that what you will be lifting isn't too heavy. Start at the lightest and work up until you find a weight that is comfortable. Again this isn't about ego; you don't need to impress anyone – just improve your health. As time goes on set little monthly goals to increase the weights you are lifting.

    c. Third, complete your workout each day and try to do all the exercises you have chosen within the prescribed time. When you are working out, keep moving as this keeps your body parts warmed up and reduces the risk of injury. You can chat and socialize after you finish training, which by the way is healthy for the brain.

    d. Fourth, on your day or days off, remain active – take a walk, climb stairs, do anything but sit on a couch, and within a couple of weeks you may not necessarily *see* a difference, but you will certainly begin to *feel* and notice a difference.

4) **Putting Our New Skill Into Practice** – By establishing a new workout routine, you will be replacing one of your old sedentary routines. This in itself will add vigor and confidence to your life. However be aware of one potential danger – that being the belief that since you are exercising, you can increase your calorie intake. Not true. While exercise does burn more calories than if you are sedentary, the amount you burn really isn't that much more. If you are looking to lose weight, the only

effective way is to reduce your calorie intake. Remember the saying beauty is only skin deep? Well exercise goes a lot deeper and you can't always see the benefits of your actions. A healthy life is within your grasp, all you need to do is put in the effort. If it's not working, be honest and revisit what you are doing. Maybe the intensity needs to be stepped up and the chatting or resting reduced.

5) **Pass It On** – Once you have established a consistent workout program and you are relatively consistent in attendance, you might want to share what you have experienced with your friends, so they too can overcome some of their pains and aches. Of course it's nice to have a training partner and a spouse can fit that bill nicely. In fact it's a great way to spend an hour together. Once the physical change catches up to the internal changes, you won't have too hard of a time convincing your friends to give it a try. Just remember, easy does it and one step at a time. Attract rather than promote, because people that preach are usually trying to convince themselves that what they are saying is true.

The Frank Experience – Physical Dimension

In my fiftieth year my first big challenge was the *Body for Life Program* – a very challenging twelve-week program that required me to train six days a week, one hour a day.

The first step of the program was to set my goals. I couldn't tell you the last time I was at 10% body fat but it was something I really wanted, so I wrote it down. For my bench press I had made a 240lb lift for 4 reps when I was about 34, so a 250lb lift didn't appear completely out of reach. Nor was a 350lb squat out of the question, as I had done 300lbs for 4 reps also at 34 years of age.

Once the goals were in place I went about my business of showing up every day and disciplining myself to stick with the program.

My first goal was to drop 11% body fat , from 21% to 10%.
Made it!
My second goal, bench press 250lbs for 6 reps – max to start was 180lbs.

Made it!
My third goal, to squat 350lbs for 6 reps – max to start was 200lbs.
Made it!

So did it work? Yes! Would I recommend this program? Not necessarily. I was so tired and wore out at the end I stopped exercising and over ate gaining back 5 kilos in the first two weeks. But that was me and you are you... maybe for you this program is perfect!

Now I enjoy more of an active lifestyle that keeps the aches and pains at bay. Again if you want to give a strenuous training program a shot, by all means feel free. After all only you know what's best for you, just don't allow it to be an excuse for quitting.

Today I like to walk everywhere I can, time permitting, and I like to lift weights three times a week. As for my intensity to live life to the fullest, I always intend to do my best, (keyword – intend – I don't always succeed, because as a fellow human I also fall prey to my innately lazy tendencies). Overall however, my competitive nature is waning, and for that I'm happy, because to be honest, my competitive ego hasn't been all that great of a friend in the past. That said, my objective now is to do the best I can at whatever I am doing and based solely upon *me*.

Lack of activity destroys the good condition of every human being, while movement and methodical physical exercise save it and preserve it.
Plato

Financial Dimension

Rising Above the Myths of Aging – Financially

UNFORTUNATELY MANY OF us have fallen trap to financial myths that have never allowed us to attain financial freedom. As with every other dimension these limiting beliefs are simply learned beliefs and are not true. The world is a place of abundance and that abundance is for you to embrace.

Here are a few financial myths that need to be tossed in the trash can.

Myth: It Takes Money to Make Money

No it doesn't! We are not dependent on those who are sitting on a mountain of money in order to make money. Sure, it usually requires an investment to make money or create wealth, however that investment doesn't necessarily need to be money. An investment can be your time, your home or an office space, an automobile, your energy, your love and passion, planning, training, practicing, or resources like your PC or Smart phone. In fact, any of these money-free investments can be exactly what it takes for you to make money.

Myth: I Can Never Do That

Yes you can and so can everyone else! You are not the only person alive with limiting beliefs that are holding you back from reaching your true potential personally and financially. It's negative beliefs that stand in the way of your real success and weaken your self-esteem. To overcome and transform negative beliefs you must first acknowledge them and accept them for what they are. As is the case with all beliefs, whether positive or negative, a limiting belief started off as a single thought in your mind in reaction to a specific event, or what you were told by your parents, or society in general. This thought was repeated often enough until it was accepted as an unchecked "truth" by your subconscious mind. In other words, limiting beliefs are a learned thought pattern – and can be unlearned and then re-programed with positive self-serving information.

Myth: I'll Never Be Rich

Who said? Once you begin to shed your limiting beliefs it will be your responsibility to adopt a wealthier mindset. Match your goals with who you are, so that your goals are not overwhelming, and you can actually imagine living them and feeling normal. If it's too much of a leap for you to believe the entire goal is possible, the entire goal will subconsciously appear impossible.

Myth: Money is the Root of All Evil

How can this statement be true? Is it not money that buys the aid for developing countries? Is it not money the pays the bills for homeless shelters. Is it not money that helps the less fortunate and supports charitable foundations? The truth is that money is not evil, nor is it good. Money is merely a medium of exchange. As Warren Buffet explains, "Of the billionaires I have known, money just brings out the basic traits in them. If they were jerks before they had money, they are simply jerks with a billion dollars."

Your Financial Dimension

"Your wealth can only grow to the extent that you do!"
T. Harv Eker

More and more people fear that as they grow older, their pensions (if they have a pension) will not cover their day-to-day expenses? They fear that their savings (if they have savings) will dissipate quickly and leave them unsure if they will be able to financially survive in their later years.

It's these fears that can stifle our quality of life, shroud us in depression and in many cases take away our desire to continue to live life positively and productively. So is there any way to remove these fears and add an element of confidence that we can live the remainder of our lives peacefully and financially independent? YES, there is. And winning a lottery is not the answer. Most lottery winners they are broke within a few short years. Why? Their financial thermostat doesn't change with the new windfall of money, so before you know it, they are right back financially where they were before they started. The key to this dimension is to adjusting your thermostat to a level that brings this dimension in balance with the other four dimensions.

As with everything in life the key is balance. Maintain balance within the 5 dimensions, remembering that if only one dimension is out of sync, it's impossible to have internal harmony. That doesn't mean you can't get by until you die – what it does mean is that once all dimensions are in sync, your life will be in harmony and inner peace will be yours.

So let's look at the financial dimension for a moment. Is it important? Certainly finances are important, but no more important than any of the other four dimensions. Rich people on their death bed would gladly give up all their money for extended good health. So what is it that we are hoping to achieve here? What is the magical monthly income number that you need to feel financial stability and secure?

How Much Money Do You Really Need?

How much money do you need each month to cover your basic expenses (mortgage, rent, utilities, transportation, insurance etc.)? Then, decide how much more money will you require each month to add some spice to your life – take a holiday, watch the occasional movie, join the gym, play a round of golf or buy a new pair of shoes.

Don't cheap out here, but don't set targets at the beginning that are unattainable and will only end up bursting your balloon, which will only provide negative self-talk an opportunity to snake its way back in and derail your potential. "See I knew it wouldn't work!" "It's pointless to try this stuff!" "There's no hope!"

An Example of Possible Monthly Expenses

NOTE: If you live in Canada or Sweden expect to pay a great deal more for everything than if you live in Peru or Thailand.

Basics Monthy Costs
Rent, Water, Power, Cable & Internet, Phone, Groceries,

Transportation,
Sub-Total - $2,000

Miscellaneous Expenses
New Clothing, Gym Membership, Holiday Savings, Miscellaneous
Expenses
Sub-Total - $200

Monthly Expense Totals - $2,200.00
Savings (savings, charity, education, 50% of total earnings
($2,200.00)
Taxes - $1,452.00

Total Monthly Earnings = $5,852.00 *(This isn't the norm this is
only an example.)*

Once you know how much money you'll need you can set your intention
and start the process of attaining it. The above budget of $5,852.00 per
month may look high or it may look low. In any case, it doesn't matter
because they're only numbers. Determine your own numbers that will
meet your needs and assist in you in feeling financially secure.

> *NOTE: The only limits you will ever face financially are those
> you impose upon yourself. If in your past you've been limited by
> financial justifications and/or excuses, it's time to let them go and
> positively readjust your financial thermostat.*

If you follow proven programs, remain focused and act consistently,
the question is not "Will you make money?" The only question will be,
"When and how much money will you make?" Financial success has
never been a matter of luck. Financial success is deciding on a plan,
sticking to the plan and doing whatever it takes to keep the plan moving
forward.

How to Attract Money

What's the point of making more money if our financial thermostat is
set low? We'll never be able to keep it. So the first thing we need to do
is re-program our beliefs and positively attract more money into our

life.

Five Steps for Reprogramming Our Financial Thermostat

- 1st - Define your goals. Again we must know where we want to end up, or how much we want to attract.
- 2nd - Reprogram your mind, with positive questions and answers. Write questions like: "Why am I capable of financial success?" Then, answer the question with a list of your positive talents and skills.
- 3rd - Think positive. What we think, we become.
- 4th - Visualize yourself already attaining your goals.
- 5th - Start a journal of gratitude. We attract our perfect reflection and if we are grateful the Universe will be grateful to us.

Learning How to Manage Money

Life with Money JARS

Most of us were never taught a system which will allow us to plan for financial freedom. Yes we've all heard the saying, "save 10% for a rainy day", but most people have never learned to live within a specific percentage of their total income.

The "money jar system" has the potential to set you on the path to financial freedom. Here are short description for each jar.

Necessity Account (NEC – 55%): The NECESSITY ACCOUNT is for managing your clients daily expenses. This jar covers their rent, mortgage, utilities, bills, taxes, food, clothes, etc., anything necessary to live – the necessities.

Financial Freedom Account (FFA – 10%): The FINANCIAL FREEDOM ACCOUNT is your client's golden goose. This jar holds the money they will use to invest in and develop their passive income streams. This money is never to be spent only reinvested. Never kill the goose.

Education Account (EDU – 10%): The EDUCATION ACCOUNT is

to be spent on education and personal growth. Investing in ourselves is essential for improving our most valuable assert – ourselves. Teach your client to invest in books, courses or anything with educational value.

Long Term Saving for Spending Account (LTSS – 10%): The LONG TERM SAVING FOR SPENDING ACCOUNT is for bigger purchases. Like a holiday, a new car, a house, etc.

Play Account (PLAY – 10%): The PLAY ACCOUNT is to be spent every month on purchases your client would consider fun activities like dinner out, getting a massage, or taking in a movie.

Give Account (GIVE – 5%): The GIVE ACCOUNT explains itself. This jar is all about giving to others. What you give is what you get. When you give money away you are sending a sign of abundance to the Universe. You are telling the Universe that you have plenty, which will magnetically ignite the law of attraction.

How to Make Additional Money

So where do you start? Well there's only really one place to start – look in the mirror and ask yourself two questions:

1. "What is my passion, something I love to do and don't need to get paid to do it?"

2. "How can I do this with a greater purpose in mind?"

That's where it all begins. It doesn't matter what you or others think is possible and it doesn't matter if there are millions of people doing it already. What matters is that *you* do it, to the best of your ability. Stick to it and do it with your greater purpose in mind. Don't underestimate the importance of the last point. When your self-defeating behavior attempts to limit you, your greater purpose will continue to drive you forward. So know that purpose, believe in that purpose and live that purpose.

Achievement of your happiness is the only moral purpose of your life, and that happiness, not pain or mindless self-indulgence, is the proof of your moral integrity, since it is the proof and the result of your loyalty to the achievement of your values.
Ayn Rand

Now let's take the time to think of some things you do well, such as:

- how to make specialty bread & buns
- how to catch a 10 pound trout
- how to color hair
- how you overcame a personal tragedy or an addiction
- how to grow a garden
- how to acquire a government grant
- how to frame a house
- how to greet customers so that they feel appreciated

The list is endless, as are your passions and expertise. Remember we all have something to share. Take a minute and think about it. What flips your switch and how could you teach it to others? It's not important that you be a "Certified Expert" to start with, because once you start teaching your knowledge will expand and the more your knowledge expands the more qualified you will become and the more expertise you will attain.

Once you lock down on your idea then you need to determine how to get paid for your expertise. Well in today's world, probably the best place to start is the internet! Now before you close the book and start freaking out about computers and the internet know this – the fastest growing demographic on the internet today are people 50 to 65 years of age.

If the internet appears terrifying, vast or complex, it's really not – it's just like anything new. Think back in your past and look for situations that initially appeared scary, but once you got your feet wet, the job or task was like second nature (a new job, driving a car, or even sex). Also keep this in mind: fears are not real; they are merely thoughts that we've engaged, given life to, added energy and then turned into our reality to keep us trapped in the same state we so desperately want to escape.

As of 2011, in the US, approximately 34 million people work from their residence and by the year 2016 close to 63 million people will work from their home.
Forrester Research, a technology and market research company.

So what does working from home mean to people who are looking for a little additional spending cash – additional cash to help make ends meet, or simply just want something to do and wouldn't mind receiving a little remuneration for their efforts? It means it's all possible for each and every one of us to add additional income at our convenience – doing what we love.

The world as we know it is changing. Every day new opportunities become available to all of us. There is a light at the end of the tunnel and if we are willing to step through our fears and become willing to educate ourselves, our financial needs can be effectively addressed from the comfort of our own home. All we need is a computer, access to the internet and enough education to give us the confidence to get the ball rolling.

As I stated in the mental dimension, our minds never shut down. The only thing that stops us from learning is our limiting beliefs (beliefs are learned and beliefs can be unlearned) and our inability to discipline ourselves to stay focused and determined in completing the task at hand.

Electronic business commonly referred to as "eBusiness" or "e-business", or an internet business, may be defined as the application of information and communication technologies (ICT) in support of all the activities of business. Commerce constitutes the exchange of products and services between businesses, groups and individuals and can be seen as one of the essential activities of any business. Electronic commerce focuses on the use of ICT to enable the external activities and relationships of the business with individuals, groups and other businesses.
http://en.wikipedia.org/wiki/E-business

Prior to embarking on this new business venture, again I remind you that we all have something of value to share with the rest of the world. It's when we are in the state of giving that we are in the reciprocal state of receiving (never will a gift received ever contain the same internal value as a gift given.) So what are some possible options for developing additional income? Or, best of all passive income?

Internet Income Options:

- Building a blog on our experiences and/or expertise
- Podcasting on our experiences and/or expertise
- Building a website to sell affiliate products
- Selling on eBay

Non-Internet Income Options:

- Sell multi-level marketing products
- Teaching English in a non-native English speaking country
- Do telemarketing and sales

Other examples of work from home jobs might include: administrative assistant (also known as virtual assistants), advertising sales agents, computer software engineer, copy editors, corporate event planner, desktop publisher, data entry clerk (be careful with this one as there have been many scams involved with data entry in the past), insurance underwriter, market research analyst, and paralegal.

Additional opportunities may include; sales representative positions, customer service representatives and online tech support for any number of industries. Then of course there's your personal experience and expertise which you can parlay into part-time or full-time online positions.

If you are so inclined, you can attend a community college course, where upon graduation you can secure a position in creative services like desktop publishing, graphic design and editing, illustration, web design and freelance writing.

Then there's turning you hobby or lifelong dream into a business by providing a consulting service.

As you can see, the options are limitless. But there are still a few myths that need to be overcome pertaining to multi-level marketing, living in third world countries and working on the internet. If you're being held back by myths and wives tales there's a very good chance that it was that type of thinking that has kept you financially restricted throughout your life. After reading the first three dimensions, you've probably recognized some of your limiting beliefs and are now willing to do some re-programming that will set you financially free.

Keep this front and center - there is absolutely nothing you or any other human can't do with the proper training and guidance. There is always a way to make it happen – you just have to keep an open mind, believe in what you are doing and keep moving in the direction of your goal.

So let's get started. Below are three avenues to make money on the internet that will require you taking the lead and running your show. As far as opportunities that will involve you working for others, I think they are self-explanatory and can be obtained through companies such as:

- www.monster.com
- www.usajobs.gov
- www.jobopenings.net

…and many others.

> *Doing what you love is the cornerstone of having abundance in your life.*
> **Wayne Dyer**

Internet Income Options

Building a Blog

The first step is to decide on a name for your blog. For those of you that struggle making a decision of any type here are a few tips to get you started:

- Keep the name short.
- Let the name reflect your intended business.
- Write a list of ten possibilities.
- Narrow it down to the top 3.

If you can't narrow it down from there write them on a piece of paper. Close your eyes and point. The closest to your finger will do. Seriously, if you struggle making a decision the inability to make a decision has obviously been a negative pattern that has held you back in the past. If making a decision was no big deal, great!

The second step is to book your domain name. Once you start you will see why you picked 10 possibilities. Chances are some of your top picks will be unavailable, even if it was simply your name. There are many websites where you can buy domain names and host your new website – such as www.bluehost.com or www.godaddy.com.

Before selecting a domain site or a server, do a little "Googling" (researching on the internet) beforehand to see what others have to say. Any additional education attained from searching has never hurt anyone!

The third step is to find a free blog or if you wish a paid blog that may even cover your hosting costs. Probably the number one choice for a blogging site is www.wordpress.com. However there are other sites like www.weebly.com and www.blogger.com that provide excellent services as well.

Once you have your blog loaded, then you're ready to begin blogging. The best way to do this is to pick specific days in which you will release your blogs so your followers know when to tune in, for example Monday and Friday or Tuesday and Thursday. Blog articles work best when they are about 400 words. Write about something you are passionate about. Write so you will engage the readers and they will want to comment back. Speak about the topic and how it can help them. Avoid self-promotion.

You must plan to keep going, because it will take time to build a following. Comment on other blogs that share the same interest. Open a Twitter account (www.twitter.com) and learn how to automatically "tweet" your blog (alert followers to new blog posts).

Once you have a solid core audience you can add additional pages to your blog and you can call them "Offer Pages". If people are interested, they will search out your products and not feel pressured to buy. Once they do buy you will want to keep these customers so you will want to build additional "Offers" with new products that will hopefully interest them.

Podcasting

Podcasting is very similar to blogging, whereas in blogging you write and in podcasting you speak. It helps if you write a little teaser text to spark interest so your viewers will want to play the podcast.

Again the first thing to do is to decide upon a name for your podcast. Again for those of you that struggle making a decision of any type follow the steps we used in the blog section. Again the name for a podcast is nowhere as important as the information you podcast delivers.

Again the second step is to book your domain name by following the same steps as the blogging section. As far as hosting goes do a little Googling beforehand to see what others have to say about the best hosts for podcasting, keeping in mind that podcasting can get expensive if you don't pay attention to your plan. Some examples of podcasting hosts are www.libsyn.com, www.podbean.com and www.buzzsprout. com

For the most part your podcasting host will provide you all the tools to get you up and running. Tools like RRS feeds, Facebook and Twitter links and the all-important feed to iTunes.

Once you have your podcast up and ready it's time to begin podcasting. Again pick a specific day or days in which to release your podcast so that your followers will know when to tune in to the show. Speak about something you are passionate about so you will engage the listeners. Acquire guests that share similar interests and speak about the topic and how it can help your audience. Go fishing for an audience and seek out people that will be kind enough to promote your podcast. Once you have a solid core audience you can add additional pages to your podcast home page and provide "Offers" to the viewers. If you get a big enough herd (followers) it's time to look for sponsors to assist you with your financial requirements.

Building a Website

Because your primary intent in building a website is to make money - NOW - you want to look around and see what it is that other money generating websites are doing. The key word here is "doing". You can take a lot of courses, read a lot of books, feel inspired, see the potentiality – and you can make all the right affirmations about attracting wealth. But unless you *take action*, nothing will change within your bank account.

As with a blog and a podcast you can sell and make money from pretty much anything on the internet, but first you need to know where to find your customers and how to attract your customers and last but certainly not least, how to convince them to buy your product.

We are all creatures of habit and tend not to stray far from the herd, no matter how different you may think you are. So the key is to take a look at how the successful internet marketers in your chosen area sell their products. Again you can't sell anything until you put something up for sale.

So whether you want to sell physical products (shoes, fishing rods, cosmetics) or you want to sell digital products (training courses, books, teaching guides) it makes no difference - just sell something you like and something that will keep you inspired and motivated. If you have your own product, great – sell it. But if you don't, it's OK to sell other people's products. This is called affiliate sales, where you put a link or a banner ad on your page that directs your customer to either a sales page or to the product supplier's page. When the product is purchased the supplier will pay you a commission for your sales.

Some websites to find affiliate programs are:

- www.commisionjunction.com
- www.affiliatetraction.ca
- www.offervault.com

...to name a few. Commissions vary from product to product so it's up to you to do your research in determining what products you will want to sell.

Selling on Ebay

Rather than duplicate eBay's efforts, visit their introductory training center for more information: http://pages.ebay.com/education

Part of your heritage in this society is the opportunity to become financially independent."
Jim Rohn

Your First Five Financial Footsteps

1) **Acceptance and Accountability** – Your first financial step should be look at your net worth. Are you happy with your financial worth? Are you happy with the amount of income you receive monthly and are you financially set up for the remainder of your life? If you cannot answer "yes" to these questions, you need to re-evaluate your financial thermostat.

   What are the beliefs that you have accepted in your life that are limiting you from allowing money to flow freely into your life? Are the phrases: money is the root of all evil, having money will turn me into a bad person and/or money creates all kinds of problems part of your past financial education? If so, you need to shed these myths and excuses and allow money to flow freely into your life by incorporating new positive beliefs.

   To be financially stable and secure is every person's right. It's time to stand up, accept why you are where you are and decide that from this day forward you will re-educate yourself as to how to balance your financial dimension.

2) **Establish Goals** – What is it that you really want and what are you willing to do to obtain it? Establish your financial needs, write them down and begin the process of obtaining them. Again develop a money management system that teaches you how to manage your money. If you can't manage a little money you will never be able to manage a lot of money.

For review again here is Jar Money Management System:

Save 10% for your financial security – this money you will never spend only re-invest
Save 10% for future investments – this money you will buy a computer or a car
Save 10% for personal growth – this money you will spend on your education
Save 10% for charity – this money you will invest in the wellbeing of others
Save 10% for fun – this money you will spend on yourself or enjoyable activities
Spend 50% on your monthly expenses

3) **Experience Your Goals** – Here is where your financial dimension begins to take on a life of its own. Here is where you start to reprogram your financial thermostat. Here is where you become aware of you past behaviors and actions and determine to put an end to those past practices that may be limiting you. From this point forward, begin putting money into each of those bank accounts and limiting your monthly spending to 50% of your take home pay. The really interesting aspect of money is that once you put your focus on it, it magically begins to appear.

Here is a little exercise that definitely works for those that have the willpower and diligence to stick with it.

Money Visualization

Visualize money coming to you. See yourself taking the mail out of your mailbox and finding checks made out to you. Imagine that your paycheck has doubled in size. Imagine money coming into your bank account from a multitude of sources. See yourself as worthy of receiving money, and visualize yourself partaking in numerous activities that you can now afford because you are financially independent.

Does having financial freedom bring you happiness?

Don't give up on this, you must change the way you see money, you must believe that it is your God given right to be financially free. Take the time to really imagine yourself financially free and all the people that you can help to have better lives. Feel the gratitude for your acts of kindness, feel the peace in your heart knowing that you are entitled to this lifestyle. That this has always been your right and now you are ready and willing to accept the responsibility of do whatever it takes to reap these rewards.

Feel it as though it's real.

Feel the joyful feelings you will have when money comes to you. Receive this money with gratitude so that those that give you this money can feel the love in giving.

4) **Putting Our New Skill Into Practice** – You can read all you want, dream all you want, but until you actively begin the process of changing your outlook and approach to money nothing will change. Starting today, and for the next 10 days, write down everything you spend money on. EVERYTHING! At the end of the 10 days, look at your list and see if there is any way to reduce spending, that will improve your money awareness, appreciation and improve your financial dimension. Become a receiver and accept money and gifts graciously. You deserve to have this dimension balance with the other 4 dimensions. You are worthy, so receive!

5) **Pass It On** – Once you get a handle on the type of work you wish to do, or new job you wish to begin, or new project you want to launch, it's time to share your newfound knowledge with others, so they too can overcome some of their fears and challenges. The other advantage of helping and teaching others is that you end up expanding your own knowledge base. Just remember as with the other dimensions, easy does it and one step at a time. Helping others to help themselves is one of the greatest gifts we can ever give to ourselves.

The Frank Experience – Financial Dimension

Twice in my life I've made a million dollars or more and twice in my life it's all gone to hell in a hand basket. Why? My financial thermostat was set incorrectly. I knew how to make it but I didn't know how to keep it or better yet I needed to get rid of it quickly because I didn't want to become an evil person. Sound familiar? Well now I know the problem encompassed more than just money. The problem was that my dimensions were out of balance. Mentally, I didn't know what to do with the money I had. Emotionally, I thought I could buy my way to happiness. Physically, I wasn't taking care of body. And spiritually, I was lost – heaven wasn't a part of my lifestyle – hell was.

But you know life works in mysterious ways and I personally believe in the biblical statement, "Ask and You Shall Receive" and here is the proof.

I was working for a friend in Thailand and he lost the contract he had hired me to complete so he had to let me go. He was a great boss and the company served a wonderful purpose within the community, so when he told me he had to let me go I just smiled, shook his hand and told him I was grateful for the opportunity.

Like I said, in the past I wasn't very good with managing money. In fact with that last paycheck before being let go, I had given most of it away. Part of my check I gave to a young student to cover university tuition. Part of my check I had given to a friend, so she could purchase a tractor/rototiller for her elderly father to make his work in the rice fields a little easier. Luckily for me I had paid my rent, but by the third week of the month, I was down to my last 20 Baht (60cents). I thought to myself, I guess it's time to test my beliefs – so I walked into a 7/11 and asked for two 10 Baht coins. I then walked out to the street and gave the coins to two people begging on the street.

It took me a couple of hours to walk home. When I got there, I sat down on my bed, set down my cell phone and said, "OK God what's next". The moment those words left my mouth my phone rang. It was a friend I hadn't spoken to in a few months. He said, "Hey I'm in town and I was wondering if I could swing by and pay you back that 8,000 Baht I borrowed from you". Coincidence you think?

Well that wasn't the first time. When my sons were 4 and 5 years of age I had booked them to sing at the children's hospital in Vancouver. I was attending college in Victoria at the time and financially we were tapped, as my student loan wasn't due to arrive for two more weeks. In fact all we had left was $25 in our overdraft account. The trip to Vancouver via the city bus and then the ferry was going to cost us $23.50 leaving me with a difficult choice. Do I go and spend the money? Or do I stay, break the little kids' hearts in Vancouver and then try and squeeze every penny I could out of the $25 over the next two weeks? Well I decided to go and again trust that my higher power would provide. To make a long story shorter, the next morning after returning from Vancouver my student loan check came in early.

Point being that money is always available and will always appear when we need it so long as we believe it's available.

In the past, my money thermostat had been set at "just get by" – a subconscious mantra I had acquired from my mother – and that's exactly what I'd done. If I had a lot of money, I gave it away or blew it to get back to comfortable and just get by. If I didn't have enough I figured out how to get just enough money to get by.

So what have I done to increase my financial thermostat? I've found a greater purpose than myself to keep me inspired until the day I die.

> *Successful people make money. It's not that people who make money become successful, but that successful people attract money. They bring success to what they do.*
> **Wayne Dyer**

Spiritual Dimension

Rising Above the Myths of Aging - Spiritually

WHEN WE LACK spirituality we feel incomplete. No matter what else happens in our life without a deeper sense of spirituality we will feel separated from others and it's that lack of connection that leaves us feeling empty and alone.

Here are a few spiritual myths that need to be tossed in the trash can.

Myth: There will always be a Separation between You and Your Higher Power

Nothing could be farther from the truth. When you live your life to the best of your ability and your actions intentionally cause no harm, your will and your Higher Power's will are one.

Myth: When you Die You will Go to Heaven or Hell

Religious beliefs are subject to the men that wrote them. And while in most cases they may have been written with good intent, they are still subject to the flaws of men. That said, Heaven and Hell are not destination points. They are a state of being. When your life is in balance and you are causing no harm to yourself or others, and you are functioning at the best of your ability, you are in the state of love, or Heaven. When you are filled with unbalanced emotions like uncertainty, anxiety and anger, you are in a state of discontent, or Hell.

Myth: Spirituality is a Religion

Spirituality is not a religion. Spirituality is a personal search for oneness with all – to find true connection with a higher power.

Myth: There is Sin

God doesn't tally wrongs. Only man does that to himself. When we get past beliefs that have been passed down to us, we come to realise that mistakes are the only possible way to grow as human beings. If our Higher Power operated on the same premise as man seeking to judge and condemn what possible hope would there be of becoming the best we can be and finding a true connection with the universe?

Your Spiritual Dimension

To accomplish great things, we must not only act, but also dream; not only plan, but also believe.
Anatole France

Spirituality, in its most narrow sense, pertains itself to matters of the spirit. Spirituality is often associated with non-physical, eternal perceptions of humankind's ultimate nature, a sense of connection with something greater than oneself such as faith or belief, which may or may not include some form of emotional experience of a perceived religious nature.

Often spiritual traditions, share a common theme: the path, practice, or tradition of understanding one's true meaning and the relationship one has with the rest of existence, a higher power, and the universe or life.

The word spirituality tends to conjure up its fair share of controversy. However, what we believe to be important is not whom you consider to be your higher power, but only that you are willing to open your mind and consider that there may be some power or force of nature that has and will continue working with you when formulating and attaining your goals and dreams.

Once you are willing to place your faith in a higher power, whether that be God, Buddha, Allah, or Mother Nature, you will be able to tap into your spiritualist dimension – which allows you access and accept miracles as they unfold in your daily life.

There are no mistakes, no coincidences. All events are blessings given to us to learn from.
Elisabeth Kubler-Ross

Upon acceptance of our spirituality, conscious awareness becomes an ever-increasing part of our lives. With that awareness comes acceptance to life, as life unfolds. When we accept life as it is, we can make adjustments that are appropriate, effective and realistic. Self-discipline becomes more prevalent and we become more aware of our responsibilities and our power of choice.

Meditation

Meditation is not about religious or philosophical beliefs. Meditation is about conscious awareness. When practicing meditation our intellectual beliefs become trivial. In meditation we seek to access our inner reality. To go beyond our conscious awareness and all the information others have told and to access the wisdom of the ages.

With expanded conscious awareness we begin to live in the "now," we begin to experience life minute-by-minute, moment-by-moment – we actually begin to live.

Eckhart Tolle has written a fascinating book called *The Power of Now* and in his book he describes the benefits of living in the now. Following is a little introduction taken from his website, www.EckhartTolle.com.

> Most people are ill at ease and restless because they are all the time bewildered by the constant inflow of thoughts in their mind. They can't stop thinking. There is no inner peace and calm. They give the impression of being haunted by something. Their emotions give rise to new thoughts and their thoughts give rise to new emotions. So they are fettered to this vicious chain of cause and effect. This is what makes them so unhappy, because they seem not to be able to let loose of their thoughts and enjoy the happiness of the Here and Now. All the time their thoughts take them adrift.
>
> For the mind creates the past and the future. If we would have no thoughts we would be forever living in the happiness of an Eternal Now. But instead, our thoughts force us to be mesmerized by our past, both with guilt and with feelings of nostalgia, and also by the future, the outcome of which is

always too uncertain and too fickle to make it worth a second thought, one would say; but nevertheless people go on thinking and worrying, which are in most cases synonymous, about the future.

Out of fear for the Void behind our thoughts we keep clinging to the content of our mind. We can not let our thoughts be for what they are, mere bubbles in a vast ocean, but we are so used to identifying our self with mind, that our whole notion of self is derived from it. We just give our mind too much credit and what is worse: we think we are having these thoughts, while it would be more accurate to say that Consciousness is having these thoughts in this particular mind in this particular body.

So in order to be happy we have to learn to disidentify with our thoughts and emotions and take a higher stance in witnessing our internal life. That way we shall develop presence in the Here and Now and learn not to be taken away anymore.

Having spent the better part of my life trying either to relive the past or experience the future before it arrives, I have come to believe that in between these two extremes is peace.
Author Unknown

Spiritual power is our ability to still make decisions with greater awareness. Spiritual power resides within us. Spiritual power is wisdom, or the ability to make decisions with maximum awareness – and to consider the ramifications of our actions before we make them. To be aware of these consequences is consciousness, and to be conscious ultimately means to accept life on life's terms. What is – is!

Awakening
An "awakening" is a moment of clarity in which a new insight or understanding is gained. With this new awareness the experience of life is seen differently, and new possibilities are opened. Changes in patterns of thought, emotions, and behavior occur. An awakening allows the possibility of growth to new levels of psychological and spiritual maturity.
lessons4living.com

It's the non-acceptance of what is, that retards spiritual growth. This non-acceptance is in actuality avoidance of accepting and dealing with pain, which we experience when facing our fears, the unknown, and situations that don't favor us. To avoid these fears, we apply subconscious defenses; we actually block or discard unpleasant facts from our awareness, thus limiting our conscious awareness.

To overcome these defenses and fully realize and embrace our potentialities, we must find the courage to accept life as it is presented to us and to accept the pain and suffering that is a necessary component of our growth. What this all boils down to is that in order to solve our problems we must solve our problems. We must honestly accept them, address them, and deal with them.

Once we commit to honestly dealing with our pain and suffering we are well on our way. Of course no one is perfect and slips will happen; however, over time our internal paradigm will begin to shift and we will be more effectively able to accept and deal with our fears.

At times this process may appear as though we are taking one step forward and two steps back. However, nothing in life of any value comes easy. That being said, everything we do to enhance any of our five dimensions will pay dividends throughout our remaining years.

Ways to Develop Our Spiritual Dimension

Meditation

Meditation allows one to still the mind and allow new insight to enter into our lives.

- ❖ Set 20 to 30 minutes aside each day – this is a great way to start your day off on a positive note.
- ❖ Find a quiet place to sit where you won't be disturbed. It's not important to sit in the lotus position; a comfortable chair will be fine. Dress comfortably.
- ❖ It's best to set an alarm so that you won't have to worry about time.
- ❖ Focus on your breath. Breathe naturally.
- ❖ Focus on your breathing and nose area. When you notice

thoughts entering your mind gently move them out of your consciousness and refocus on your breathing.

❖ When your time is up slowly open your eyes, take a few deep breaths, and stand up slowly.

Most people have trouble letting go of the Western world's tendency to think, think and think some more. To think is only rehashing old information. Be patient; a turbulent mind will take time to be tamed.

Meditative techniques play an important role in the Arthritis Self-Help Course at Stanford University. Fifteen to twenty percent of the more than 100,000 people with arthritis that took the 12-hour course and learned the meditation-style relaxation exercises reported a reduction in pain.

A strong link has also been established between the practice of Transcendental Meditation and longevity. Only two factors have been scientifically determined to actually extend life: caloric restriction and lowering of the body's core temperature. Meditation has been shown to lower core body temperature.
http://www.1stholistic.com

Ying and Yang Therapy Balls

Therapy balls are made of various metals and can be painted in a multitude of designs and colors. The balls are delicately weighted and at times may encompass soothing chimes. According to traditional Chinese beliefs, our vital organs are all connected to the fingers. By rotating these balls in one hand it is believed that this action stimulates the circulation of blood and energy throughout the body.

Prayer

Prayer is the act of attempting to communicate, commonly with a sequence of words, with a deity or spirit for the purpose of worshiping, requesting guidance, requesting assistance, confessing sins, or to express one's thoughts and emotions. The words of the prayer may take the form of a hymm, incantation, or a spontaneous utterance in the praying person's words.
Wikipedia

For decades the medical community basically ignored the impact of religion on health. But in recent years, scientists have begun studying

the possibility that faith matters. "There are hundreds and hundreds of studies – scientific studies – that show that religious people are healthier."
Dr. Harold Koenig, Duke University's Center for Spirituality, Theology and Health.

Prayer can be a very effective way to relieve oneself of stress and anxiety. When we pray we surrender control over a situation and ask for help. The act of asking for help opens the door and allows the universe to assist us. The challenge is to keep an open mind and the awareness to see the answers to our prayers, as they may not resemble exactly what we had asked for. In fact they may be better!

St. Frances Prayer

Lord, make me an instrument of thy peace!
That where there is hatred, I may bring love.
Where there is wrong, I may bring the spirit of forgiveness.
That where there is discord, I may bring harmony.
That where there is error, I may bring truth.
That where there is doubt, I may bring faith.
That where there is despair, I may bring hope.
That where there are shadows, I may bring light.
That where there is sadness, I may bring joy.
Lord, grant that I may seek rather to comfort, than to be comforted.
To understand, than to be understood.
To love, than to be loved.
For it is by self-forgetting that one finds.
It is by forgiving that one is forgiven.

There are two sayings that have the potential to lead us to miracles, (Faith Can Move Mountains and No Prayer Goes Unanswered) yet there are those of us who are still reluctant and skeptical to believe. But why? What possible harm can come of us if we exercise faith? By exercising faith all things are possible, without faith we are limited, limited to our perceived limitations.

A father walked into his son's room while the little boy was praying.
"Son, why do you knee and pray? Praying is a waste of time." The little boy looked up and said "God answers my prayers."
The father shook his head and said, "There is no God, you are wasting

your time."

The little boy again looked up at his Dad and said, "There is a God and he answers my prayers."

The father shot back, "Oh really, well you've been praying for a new bike for over a year now

and I don't see any bike out there, so tell me how did God answer that prayer."

The little boy smiled and said, "Not yet."

Author Unknown

Everything in life has its time and place. We as humans tend to focus on our immediate needs and wants, limiting our view of life as a whole. However the more we practice our spirituality, the more positive our approach is to life's daily challenges, trials, and tribulations that we begin to see life as it truly is, amazing and abundant.

Your First Five Spiritual Footsteps

1) **Acceptance and Accountability** – How could we ever believe in something we cannot see? Well there's always electricity or oxygen. We don't dispute their existence and we can't see them either. So why do so many of us dispute spiritually and the existence of a higher power? Probably because our ego doesn't like the competition, our egos want us to believe we are the masters of our own destiny, that we are our own Gods. In part this belief is true, but like thinking (rehashing ours or others old thoughts over and over) why would we want to limit ourselves when the rewards are so amazing? Every day we are presented with countless miracles that we blow off as coincidences or the norm.

   Most often, because we are too stressed or going way too fast to ever notice. The key is to open our minds to the endless possibilities that are presented to us daily. Miracles are happening every moment. It is our acceptance of a higher power and the coinciding gift of humility that allows us to see and reap the benefits of these miracles. In life what we give we get. So if we want happiness and peace, we need to be sure that's what we are putting out to the universe.

2) **Establish Goals** – When we develop goals in our spiritual dimension, it is very important that we have a greater plan in mind. It's one thing to set a goal to make a million dollars; it's a completely different thing to set a goal to make a million dollars with the intent of helping others while helping yourself. When we are thinking spirituality, our limits are endless as to what we may set for goals. This is the dimension where miracles are designed and manifested. In this dimension we need to understand that everything is possible. Positive belief and faith returns positive results, negative beliefs return negative results. So if you set no limits upon your thoughts – you in turn set no limits upon your reality.

Physical Reality is a Manifestation of Thoughts
They have demonstrated what the "New Science" has been pointing to for nearly half a century: that our universe is more like a thought than a thing and is actually a manifestation of consciousness. While this will be one of science's most life-changing revelations ever, for many it will not be a new notion ... just as the spherical nature of the earth and the sun's central place in our universe were not new ideas once they were finally accepted by the masses.

The truth of the creative nature of thought has also been around for a very long time. Mostly, it's been known in the domain of religion and spirituality - "As ye believe, so shall it be," "We reap what we sow." However, in 2004, filmmaker and entrepreneur William Arntz brought these ideas - and their scientific underpinnings - to millions more through his groundbreaking, award-winning, hybrid documentary feature film, What the BLEEP Do We Know!? The film explored the emerging convergence of these ancient spiritual principles with leading edge science. And pointed out how adherence to these new notions of reality will utterly change the planet.
By Thomas Herold in Scientific Background on March 2nd, 2007
www.dreammanifesto.com

3) **Experience Your Goals** – Again, there are no short cuts in attaining our spiritual goals. Spiritual growth comes with spiritual practice. If we stick to it we will soon realize just how much more positive our life is becomes.

   a. First, ensure that we really believe in what we want to attain. That our goal aligns with our core beliefs of who we are and what we really want to do. Just because Joe has it doesn't mean it's what you want.

b. Second, let go of our goal. If the goal is of a worthy cause it will now manifest itself all by itself. It is our job to go about the daily business of living our lives in the now and doing the next right thing to help our goal materialize.

c. Third, be aware of the signposts that are presented to us as we embark upon this journey. Through our increased awareness our higher power provides the guidance, but it's up us to walk through the door and get the job done.

During a terrible flood a man was seen hanging out of his 2nd story window by two would be rescuers in a boat. "Quick jump in the boat!" one of the rescuers cried. "It's OK, God will save me." The man replied. A couple of hours passed and the water continued to rise. The man had now climbed on the roof and was spotted by a rescue helicopter. "Quick grab the rope!" the pilot called out over the P.A. system. "It's OK, God will save me." The man replied. A couple of hours passed and to the man's surprise the man found himself standing at the gates of heaven. He looked up at God and said, "Why didn't you save me?" God replied, "Who do you think sent the boat and the helicopter?"

4) **Putting Our New Skill Into Practice** – Discipline, discipline, and more discipline. Sorry but again nothing of any value comes easy in life. Meditation and prayer take time to get a handle on.

First let's look at meditation. Meditation takes time to reach a point where it becomes productive and when we are able to quell our monkey minds for more than a few seconds (There's an endless battle that rages between our ears, engaging the past and our perceived future). It is very important that we be patient with ourselves, and that we try to be as consistent as possible when we practice. Remember we don't need to be perfect; we just need to give this new skill set a fair chance. In fact it may be a good idea to take in a mediation workshop.

When we address prayer, we are referring to prayer as sending out a positive message into the universe with the intent of making the world a better place. So when we pray, it only makes sense to send love through pray for others. If we have faith we don't need to pray for ourselves; our higher power has that all under control. Live the old saying "what we give, we get."

5) **Pass It On** – As our manifestations become reality, those closest to us will witness our shift in attitude and demeanor. Keep in mind that throughout our spiritual journey more will be revealed to us daily on a need to know basis. Again the key is to share what we have experienced, not what we have read. We only want to put it out there for others, so they can decide for themselves if this is what they want. When people are ready to learn their teacher will appear, all we can do is plant the seed.

The Frank Experience – Spiritual Dimension

I've been blessed with a number of truly amazing experiences in my life; however, none more impressive or enlightening than the one that happened about twelve years ago in Nashville, Tennessee.

Five years after my sons' eventful summer of singing on the Victoria causeway, they found themselves signing a major label recording contract with Polydor Records in Nashville. While living in Nashville we would take the opportunity to, once a month, sing at the children's hospital.

During one of those visits after the boys had performed, I asked the hospital's PR representative if there were any shut-ins, and if we could possibly go to their room to sing them a song or two. Sure enough, there were a couple. After singing to the two children, we were walking down the hall on our way out of the hospital, and I noticed a little girl about three or four years old lying in a bed.

I asked the nurse if we could sing for her. She said she didn't think it was a good idea, because the little girl only had a couple of weeks left to live. I didn't always have my emotions in check, so I proceeded to say with a somewhat challenging tone, "Well, ask the mom?" The nurse refused, and my voice began to rise as I said, "If she only has two weeks left why do you want to prevent her from experiencing something so positive and uplifting?"

Just then, the doctor walked by and asked what the problem was. After I explained, the doctor offered to ask the little girl's mother. Thankfully, the mother invited us in.

The boys introduced themselves to this frail little girl and proceeded to sing a song on their album that Garth Brooks had written: "When God Made You." Everyone broke into tears. Then the boys sang a little ditty that Clint (one of the triplets) and I had written called: "With a Little Smile." Then everyone was back to smiling.

As we were leaving the room, I realized I had one of the boy's CD's with me, so I went back and asked her if she would like it. She nodded and I gave it to her. I then told her that we were going out on the road to sing, but if she was there when we got back in four weeks, I would give her the boy's other CD.

When we got back off of the road, I had the record label book us another show at the hospital. After the show we walked down to her ward to see if she was still there, CD in hand. We had just opened the doors to the ward and the head nurse came over to us and said, "Mr. Moffatt, she's been asking for that CD every day since you guys left."

She had made it past the two weeks, so I came up with another idea. I told her that in two months the boys would be doing a show with Toby Keith, in downtown Nashville – and that if she could get strong enough to leave the hospital, I would get her front row tickets to the concert. Two months later she was sitting front row.

After that show we headed out to Las Vegas and didn't get back until November. When we returned to Nashville, we had the record label again schedule a show at the hospital, and after the show we went straight to her ward. When we got there the nurse we spoke to said she was gone. Our hearts all dropped, and she then realized what she had said and corrected herself saying, "No, no she's gone home."

After that we moved to Las Vegas, Nevada, and then to Branson,

Missouri, and then spent five years touring the world. We never saw that little girl again, but we learned a very valuable lesson – she believed, when others didn't, and she survived. She is a miracle.

Every day we are all witnesses to miracles, some small, some incredible. I've learned to accept them for what they are and not try to intellectualize them away. Now I work at accepting life as it unfolds each day. I've taken my turn at playing God in my life, (challenging others to do things my way, because I knew what was best for them) but to be honest I didn't do a very good job of it. So from here on out, I think I'll just try and follow my higher power's queue and respect others to make their own best decisions and choices.

> *When we look for love and acceptance from another being it is only to fill*
> *the void and emptiness we have failed to fulfill within ourselves.*
> **Frank Moffatt**

Conclusion

S O NOW IT'S up to you. The door has been opened and you've been shown the path. What you make of it will depend 100% upon your willingness to overcome your previous beliefs and behaviors and a willingness to grow as a person in their second fifty.

The challenge here is to live your second fifty years of your life one day at a time and to the best of your ability. Once you set your dimensional targets, change will begin and over time evolution and progress is certain to happen. Remember you are human. Error and slips are just a part of the course. Be kind to yourself, forgive yourself, and then get back at it – everything is just a matter of practice, time, and effort.

Again, this isn't about coming in first, it isn't about being better than someone else, and it isn't about the final destination. This is all about the journey, all about enjoying life to its fullest, all about accepting the cards that are dealt to us, and all about making positive adjustments that lead to positive personal growth and change. There are no time limits.

If before putting *Your Second Fifty* into action you could remember one person's name out of ten – and after a month of expanding and working on your mental dimension, you were able to remember two names out of ten, well that's progress. The key to personal growth in all of the dimensions is not to compare ourselves with others or the expectations of others but to see our improvements and to be proud of them, no matter how small or how insignificant.

I wrote *Your Second Fifty* with hopes to stimulate your interests in all five dimensions of your life and with the desire that you would then make positive changes. Research, explore, and experience whatever it is that will ignite your passion within. Your second fifty years can be and should be both rewarding and productive.

At times western culture tends to disregard the value of wisdom that only comes with age. So never underestimate your value to future generations and all the wonderful benefits that they will reap from your discipline and dedication in living your second fifty years to the fullest of your potential.

> *In life we do not have the right to complain or blame. If we complain or blame we are not being accountable and responsible for our current state of affairs. Once we become accountable and responsible we receive the right to all that is ours to avail and enjoy – happiness, love, and freedom.*

Frank Moffatt

Fifty Fantastic Days

Day # 1

Fitness Facts

With any exercise program, seniors should see a doctor and obtain clearance prior to beginning the program.

Spiritual Quote

Truth, like surgery, may hurt, but it cures. **Han Suyin**

Quote of the Day

Do not believe in anything simply because you have heard it.
Do not believe in anything simply because it is spoken and rumoured by many.
Do not believe in anything simply because it is found written in your religious books.
Do not believe in anything merely on the authority of your teachers and elders.
Do not believe in traditions because they have been handed down for many generations.
But after observation and analysis, when you find that anything agrees with reason and is conducive to the good and benefit of one and all, then accept it and live up to it. **Buddha**

Food Facts

You cannot lose weight using Low Fat Diets. Low fat foods have been popular for more than 15 years, but yet our society is getting more overweight as each year passes. This fact should tell you that eating a low fat menu is not the answer to losing weight.

Mind Massage

What's filled in the morning and emptied at night,
and one day of the year its emptied in the morning
and emptied at night?

Emotional

In a book called *The Fifth Discipline* (by Peter M. Senge), Senge quotes an article called "Advanced Maturity," by B. O'Brien: "Whatever the reasons, we do not pursue emotional development with the same intensity with which we pursue physical and intellectual development. This is all the more unfortunate because full emotional development offers the greatest degree of leverage in attaining our full potential."

Money Mastery

If you want to know what God thinks of money, just look at the people he gave it to.
Dorothy Parker

Day # 2

Fitness Facts

Begin your exercise program at a relatively moderate level of intensity, progressing gradually to safely allow your body the time to adapt to the program.

Spiritual Quote

Wisdom is not a question of learning facts with the mind; it can only be acquired through perfection of living. **N. Sri Ram**

Quote of the Day

When your work speaks for itself, don't interrupt. **Henry J. Kaiser**

Food Facts

Carrots really do help prevent blindness. Vitamin A is known to prevent "night blindness," and carrots are loaded with Vitamin A.

Mind Massage

A bus driver was going down a street. He was on the wrong side. He went past a stop sign. He didn't signal at a turn. He went under the minimum speed and yet he didn't get in trouble for his actions.
Why not?

Emotion

The key to success is to keep growing in all areas of life - mental, emotional, spiritual, as well as physical. **Julius Erving**

Money Mastery

A Penny Saved is a Penny Earned **Benjamin Franklin**

Day # 3

Fitness Facts

Just because you have begun to exercise doesn't mean you can over eat during your day. If you consume more calories than you burn off in a day, you will gain weight. The key is a balanced diet and exercise plan.

Spiritual Quote

There can be no happiness if the things we believe in are different from the things we do. **Freya Madeline Stark**

Quote of the Day

To be 70 years young is sometimes far more cheerful and hopeful than to be 40 years old. **Oliver Wendell Holmes**

Food Facts

Fast food eaters can become chemically dependent on the fat and sugar found in fast food. Scientists say these substances affect the same areas of the brain as people with drug addiction.

Mind Massage

What are the next two letters in the following sequence?
E, O, E, R, E, X, ?,?

Emotion

Awfulizing: The belief that a situation is more than 100% worse than it is. Catastrophizing: Making mountains out of mole hills. **John W. Maag**

Money Mastery

Too many people spend money they earned..to buy things they don't want..to impress people that they don't like. **Will Rogers**

Day # 4

Fitness Facts

Physical activity builds physical vitality. With every year of your life, you have more to gain from being physically active.

Spiritual Quotes

People only see what they are prepared to see. **Ralph Waldo Emerson**

Quote of the Day

Dignity consists not in possessing honours, but in the consciousness that we deserve them. **Aristotle**

Food Facts

Hens with white feathers and white ear lobes produce white-shelled eggs and hens with red feathers and red earlobes produce brown eggs; the colour has no relationship to the nutritional quality or taste of the eggs.

Mind Massage

A man is at a river with a 9-gallon bucket and a 4-gallon bucket. He needs exactly 6 gallons of water. How can he use both buckets to get exactly 6 gallons of water? Note that he cannot estimate by dumping some of the water out of the 9-gallon bucket or the 4-gallon bucket.

Emotion

We can't solve problems by using the same kind of thinking we used when we created them. **Albert Einstein**

Money Mastery

There is only one class in the community that thinks more about money than the rich, and that is the poor. **Oscar Wilde**

Day # 5

Fitness Facts

Crunches and other abdominal exercises can help you strengthen your abdominal muscles and improve your posture and abdominal muscle tone. But muscle is muscle and fat is fat. If you want a more athletic waist, you need to lose the fat to show off your abdominal muscles.

Spiritual Quotes

Success isn't permanent, and failure isn't fatal. **Mike Ditka**

Quote of the Day

It's never too late to be who you might have been. **George Eliot**

Food Facts

In 1295 when Marco Polo returned from China to his homeland of Italy, he brought back a recipe for "Milk Ice." Europeans substituted cream for the milk and the dessert favourite ice-cream was born.

Mind Massage

Recently, Snow White's seven dwarfs met up with three of their friends and went to the cinema to see Bambi. From the clues below, can you determine the order in which they stood in the ticket queue?

Grumpy was in front of Dopey. Stumpy was behind Sneezy and Doc. Doc was in front of Droopy and Happy. Sleepy was behind Stumpy, Smelly, and Happy. Happy was in front of Sleepy, Smelly, and Bashful. Bashful was behind Smelly, Droopy, and Sleepy. Sneezy was in front of Dopey. Smelly was in front of Grumpy, Stumpy, and Sneezy. Dopey was in front of Droopy. Sleepy was in front of Grumpy and Bashful. Dopey was behind Sneezy, Doc, and Sleepy. Stumpy was in front of Dopey. Smelly was behind Doc.

Emotion

Most people don't realize that it is the meaning they assign to people and events that actually generates emotions. Commonly used statements such as "He made me mad." "She made me sad." or "That really made me happy." not only reflect this mistaken belief but actually reinforces it.

Money Mastery

Money isn't everything...but it ranks right up there with oxygen. **Rita Davenport**

Day # 6

Fitness Facts

Exercise can slow down, halt, and possibly even reverse many aging trends. Much of the decline that is commonly associated with the aging process is often the result of lifelong inactivity and improper lifestyle habits. Research clearly demonstrates that if an active lifestyle is maintained into later years, a relatively high level of function may be retained and vigorous activity can be engaged in both safely and successfully.

Spiritual Quotes

Begin at once to live, and count each separate day as a separate life. **Seneca**

Quote of the Day

Use what talents you possess: the woods would be very silent if no birds sang there except those that sang best. **Henry Van Dyke**

Food Facts

A North American Indian named George Crum invented potato crisps.

Mind Massage

What does this say: merepeat

Emotion

Painful as it may be, a significant emotional event can be the catalyst for choosing a direction that serves us - and those around us - more effectively. Look for the learning. **Louisa May Alcott**

Money Mastery

The man who damns money has obtained it dishonorably; the man who respects it has earned it. **Ayn Rand**

Day # 7

Fitness Facts

Weight lifting helps maintain adequate muscular strength, endurance, and tone as well as promoting joint mobility and increased flexibility.

Spiritual Quotes

I learned that we can do anything, but we can't do everything... at least not at the same time. So think of your priorities not in terms of what activities you do, but when you do them. Timing is everything. **Dan Millman**

Quote of the Day

Life is like a rose; you can lie upon the pedals or become entangled amongst the thorns. **Frank Moffatt**

Food Facts

Almonds are a member of the peach family.

Mind Massage

There is a family party consisting of two fathers, two mothers, two sons, one father-in-law, one mother-in-law, one daughter-in-law, one grandfather, one grandmother, and one grandson.

What is the minimum number of persons required so that this is possible?

Emotion

Controlling ones emotions through Doc Lew Childre's Freeze Frame technique.
1. Recognize your stressful feelings and make the decision to freeze-frame (call a time-out).
2. Shift your focus away from your racing thoughts and emotions.
3. Think about a fun time in your life; a time in which you felt positive.
4. Ask your heart for a more efficient and effective response to the situation you are freeze-framing.
5. Open yourself up and listen to the answer your heart gives you.

Money Mastery

There is nothing like a dream to create the future. **Victor Hugo**

Day # 8

Fitness Facts

Eating a low-salt, reduced fat, diet with plenty of fruits, vegetables, and fibre can actually reduce your age-related risks of heart disease, diabetes, stroke, osteoporosis, and other chronic diseases.

Spiritual Quotes

To be wise is to live in an inner harmony that eventually overcomes all outer discords. **N. Sri Ram**

Quote of the Day

We all have the extraordinary coded within us, waiting to be released. **Jean Houston**

Food Facts

Chewing gum stimulates signals in the learning centre of the brain and thus helps save memory as you age.

Mind Massage

How many letters are in the alphabet?

Emotion

In *Emotional Intelligence*, Daniel Goleman describes the five major components: **Component 1** - Knowing our emotions. Self-awareness – recognizing a feeling as it happens – is the keystone of emotional intelligence.... [T]he ability to monitor feelings from moment to moment is crucial to psychological insight and self-understanding. An inability to notice our true feelings leaves us at their mercy. People with greater certainty about their feelings are better pilots of their lives, having a surer sense of how they really feel about personal decisions from whom to marry to what job to take.

Money Mastery

It's easier to feel a little more spiritual with a couple of bucks in your pocket. **Craig Ferguson**

Day # 9

Fitness Facts

No matter how poor your current level of fitness, you can start an exercise routine and become fitter and healthier at any age.

Spiritual Quotes

The Vietnamese are our brothers; the Russians are our brothers; the Chinese are our brothers and one day we've got to sit down together at the table of brotherhood. **Martin Luther King, Jr.**

Quote of the Day

... happiness gives us the energy which is the basis of health. **Henri-Frederic Amiel**

Food Facts

Corn Flakes are about 8% corn.

Mind Massage

This engulfing thing is strange indeed, the greater it grows the less you see. What is it?

Emotion

In *Emotional Intelligence*, Daniel Goleman describes the five major components: **Component 2** - Managing emotions. Handling feelings so they are appropriate is an ability that builds on self-awareness.... People who are poor in [the ability to soothe oneself, to shake off rampant anxiety, gloom, or irritability] are constantly battling feelings of distress, while those who excel in it can bounce back far more quickly from life's setbacks and upsets.

Money Mastery

Not all dreamers are winners, but all winners are dreamers. Your dream is the key to your future. The Bible says that, "without a vision (dream), a people perish." You need a dream, if you're going to succeed in anything you do. **Mark Gorman**

Day # 10

Fitness Facts

About 25 percent of North American adults - and an even greater percentage of women - are sedentary. After age 44, upwards of 30 percent of women are sedentary, and by age 65, the proportion increases to almost 35 percent. By the time they reach age 75, about 50 percent of all women are sedentary.

Spiritual Quotes

Be kind, for everyone you meet is fighting a hard battle. **Plato**

Quote of the Day

Happiness is not a station you arrive at, but a manner of traveling. **Margaret Lee Runbeck**

Food Facts

Fortune cookies are not from China; they were invented in Los Angeles around 1920.

Mind Massage

A certain street has 1000 buildings. A sign-maker is contracted to number the houses from 1 to 1000. How many zeros will he need?

Emotion

In *Emotional Intelligence*, Daniel Goleman describes the five major components: **Component 3** - Motivating oneself. Marshalling emotions in the service of a goal is essential for paying attention, for self-motivation and mastery, and for creativity. Emotional self-control – delaying gratification and stifling impulsiveness – underlies accomplishment of every sort. And being able to get into the "flow" state enables outstanding performance of all kinds. People who have this skill tend to be more highly productive and effective in whatever they undertake.

Money Mastery

Money speaks sense in a language all nations understand. **Aphra Behn**

Day # 11

Fitness Facts

In addition to its many positive physical benefits, regular exercise can develop self-awareness of the body and improved mental well-being.

Spiritual Quotes

Wanting to reform the world without discovering one's true self is like trying to cover the world with leather to avoid the pain of walking on stones and thorns. It is much simpler to wear shoes. **Ramana Maharshi**

Quote of the Day

A man should not leave this earth with unfinished business. He should live each day as if it was a pre-flight check. He should ask each morning, am I ready to lift-off? **Diane Frolov and Andrew Schneider**

Food Facts

Fish consumption may be more than just brain food because it also helps to protect your eyes from age-related macular degeneration, which is a potential cause of blindness.

Mind Massage

One barrel of pickles weighs 60 kgs, while one box of mangoes weighs 18 kgs. What is the weight of one crate of cherries and one sack of potatoes, when the sack of potatoes and the box of mangoes together weigh as much as the barrel of pickles and the crate of cherries? Note that two crates of cherries weigh as much as one box of mangoes.

Emotion

In *Emotional Intelligence*, Daniel Goleman describes the five major components: **Component 4** - Recognizing emotions in others. Empathy, another ability that builds on emotional self-awareness, is the fundamental "people skill." People who are empathic are more attuned to the subtle social signals that indicate what others need or want. This makes them better at callings such as the caring professions, teaching, sales, and management.

Money Mastery

When you do what you fear most, then you can do anything. **Stephen Richards**

Day # 12

Fitness Facts

Men who exercise regularly are less likely to have problems with erectile dysfunction than are men who don't exercise, especially as they get older.

Spiritual Quote

The bond that links your true family is not one of blood, but of respect and joy in each other's life. **Richard Bach**

Quote of the Day

When a friend is in trouble, don't annoy him by asking if there is any thing you can do. Think up something appropriate and do it. **Edgar Watson Howe**

Food Facts

Mayonnaise will kill lice and also condition your hair.

Mind Massage

There is a one-floor house, and everything in it is blue, green or purple. The people are purple, the carpeting is green, and the walls are blue.
What colour do you suppose the stairs are?

Emotion

In *Emotional Intelligence*, Daniel Goleman describes the five major components: **Component 5** -The art of relationships is, in large part, a skill in managing emotions in others. ...These are the abilities that undergird popularity, leadership, and interpersonal effectiveness. People who excel in these skills do well at anything that relies on interacting smoothly with others; they are social stars."

Money Mastery

It is a kind of spiritual snobbery that makes people think they can be happy without money. **Albert Camus**

Day # 13

Fitness Facts

Heart disease, stroke, diabetes, osteoporosis, and cancer are all believed to be exacerbated by your lifestyle.

Spirituality

For every sin but the killing of time there is forgiveness. **Sufism**

Quote of the Day

He who is drowned is not troubled by the rain. **Chinese Proverb**

Food Facts

Heinz Catsup leaves the bottle traveling at 40 kilometres per year.

Mind Massage

A woman has 7 children, half of them are girls.
How can this be possible?

Emotion

The greater the feeling of inferiority that has been experienced, the more powerful is the urge to conquest and the more violent the emotional agitation. **Alfred Adler**

Money Mastery

You can be happy with money and you can be wretched with it. It depends on what kind of person you are. **Taylor Caldwell**

Day # 14

Fitness Facts

Older adults require exercise as much as younger individuals; however, the benefits for seniors are even more pronounced.

Spiritual Quotes

If you and I are having a single thought of violence or hatred against anyone in the world at this moment, we are contributing to the wounding of the world. **Deepak Chopra**

Quote of the Day

It is no use to blame the looking glass if your face is awry. **Nikolai Gogol**

Food Facts

Pizza originated in the early 1700's in Naples, Italy.

Mind Massage

Mr. Smith lives at 20, Rose Street with his wife Debi. They have nine sons and each son has one sister.

How many members are in Mr. Smith's family?

Emotion

Demandingness: The use of the words "should/shouldn't," "have to," "need to," and "must." These words represent a magical way to change reality to the way we want it. **John W. Maag**

Money Mastery

Money is like manure; it's not worth a thing unless it's spread around encouraging young things to grow. **Thornton Wilder**

Day # 15

Fitness Facts

Following your exercise sessions, if you don't allow the muscles adequate time to recover, you may run the risk of over training and possible injury.

Spiritual Quotes

All of us have the capacity to attract to ourselves what seems to be missing in our lives. **Dr. Wayne Dyer**

Quote of the Day

When you cease to make a contribution, you begin to die. **Eleanor Roosevelt**

Food Facts

Milk is the new diet drink since low-fat, high-calcium dairy foods may burn off fat since extra calcium increases metabolism.

Mind Massage

A person travels on a bicycle from home to church on a straight road with wind against him. He took 4 hours to reach there. On the way back to the home, he took 3 hours to reach as wind was in the same direction. If there is no wind, how much time does he take to travel from home to church?

Emotion

Once you learn and accept that emotional responses are preceded by automatic thoughts, it becomes easy to teach yourself how to focus your attention on them during the heat of the moment. Once this happens you will see for yourself that these thoughts and images appear between the events and our emotional responses.

Money Mastery

Poverty: a temporary financial low, curable by money. **Stephen Richards**

Day # 16

Fitness Facts

Moderate activity that lasts less than an hour may reduce your appetite for an additional hour or two, while intense exercise of an hour or more may increase appetite.

Spiritual Quotes

What we think, we become. **Buddha**

Quote of the Day

One's dignity may be assaulted, vandalized and cruelly mocked, but cannot be taken away unless it is surrendered. **Michael J. Fox**

Food Facts

Puffed grain was invented by Alexander Anderson in 1902. Unlike popcorn, a type of corn that naturally pops or puffs up with heat, puffed cereal or snacks are formed by exploding whole grain kernels under high pressure and steam.

Mind Massage

A boy goes into a shop to buy some sweets. He uses a $1 coin and buys 40 cents worth of sweets. The shop assistant gives him two coins for his change.
One of them was not a 50-cent piece, so how could the boy have gotten his exact change?

Emotion

Many people believe that they are powerless; that it is external circumstances that hold the power over them; that their life is simply a series or reactions against or responses to the circumstances that they encounter. In order to regain power, a person needs to believe that he or she can make choices independent of the circumstances.

Money Mastery

The lack of money is the root of all evil. **Mark Twain**

Day # 17

Fitness Facts

Muscle will never turn into fat. Muscle is muscle and fat is fat. They are two separate types of tissue.

Spiritual Quotes

The danger is that every religion, including the Catholic one, says "I have the ultimate truth." Then you start to rely on the priest, the mullah, the rabbi, or whoever, to be responsible for your acts. In fact, you are the only one who is responsible. **Paulo Coelho**

Quote of the Day

Health is not valued till sickness comes. **Dr. Thomas Fuller**

Food Facts

Strawberries are the only fruit which has its seeds on its outer skin.

Mind Massages

Five horses ran in the race. There were no ties.
Whisper did not come first. Lightning was neither first nor last.
Eclipse Glory came in one place after Whisper.
Thunder was not second.
Sunshine was two places below Thunder.
In what order did the horses finish?

Emotion

Essi Systems of San Francisco has found that only factor which does have a significant impact on a person's ability to handle stress – particularly work pressure – is personal power; i.e., control over your time, resources, information, and other elements connected with work. Says Esther Orioli, the founder of Essi Systems, "Our testing revealed that out of 21 stress-related factors we examined, personal power was the only factor that could predict who got sick and who stayed healthy in work situations with high amounts of pressure. Conversely, people without this sense of personal power tended to feel victimized and were unable to cope with high amounts of pressure in similar situations."

Money Mastery

To dream by night is to escape your life. To dream by day is to make it happen.
Stephen Richards

Day # 18

Fitness Facts

Simply adding movement into your daily routine can increase your level of fitness. Take the stairs, park so you are forced to walk, even taking the dog for a walk all counts. Try and keep tabs so that you put in 30 minutes of exercise a day.

Spiritual Quotes

The more you have, the more you are occupied, the less you give. **Mother Teresa**

Quote of the Day

I don't know the key to success, but the key to failure is trying to please everybody. **Bill Cosby**

Food Facts

Popsicles were invented by an 11 year old, Frank Epperson, when he left a stirring stick in his soda water drink overnight on his porch.

Mind Massage

You have two jars, 50 red marbles and 50 blue marbles. A jar will be picked at random, and then a marble will be picked from the jar. You can place maximum of 50 marbles in each jar.

Placing all of the marbles in the jars, how can you maximize the chances of a red marble being picked? What are the exact odds of getting a red marble using your scheme?

Emotion

Just as physical fitness exercises strengthen the body, one can strengthen ones Emotional Fitness through daily meditation and deep breathing exercises. The exercises will help strengthen your ability to deal with life's daily stresses and pains.

Money Mastery

It is not the creation of wealth that is wrong, but the love of money for its own sake. **Margaret Thatcher**

Day # 19

Fitness Facts

Taking higher amounts vitamins and supplements will not enhance you physical goals.

Spiritual Quotes

Even as the fingers of the two hands are equal, so are human beings equal to one another. No one has any right, nor any preference to claim over another. **Muhammad**

Quote of the Day

Youth is a disease from which we all recover. **Dorothy Fulheim**

Food Facts

Peanuts are one of the ingredients in dynamite.

Mind Massage

There was a crime scene at this house where a man lies dead slumped over his desk. There was a note next to him that said to push the play button. When the cops arrived they pushed it and a voice said, "My life is too complicated and I can't take it any more." Then there was a gunshot. How did the cops know that this was a murder?

Emotional

One of the most critical aspects of gaining more emotional control is to learn how to identify your automatic thoughts. In most instances, our negative emotional responses are directly preceded by automatic thoughts. These automatic thoughts remain hidden for most of us. Unless you train yourself to look for these thoughts, you will probably not be aware of them. But once you do learn how to catch hold of your automatic thoughts, you will not only become aware of them, but you also learn how to control them.

Money Mastery

If saving money is wrong, I don't want to be right! **William Shatner**

Day # 20

Fitness Facts

Only take salt tablets under a doctor's supervision. You will never sweat enough during regular exercise to require additional salt.

Spiritual Quote

Love one another. **Jesus of Nazareth**

Quote of the Day

Where there is an open mind, there will always be a frontier. **Charles F. Kettering**

Food Facts

White chocolate is not a true chocolate because it contains no chocolate; instead, it's made of sugar, cocoa butter, milk solids, lecithin, and vanilla.

Mind Massage

What row of numbers comes next?
This is a tough one!
1
11
21
1211
111221
312211
13112221

Emotion

Curiosity doesn't matter any more. These days people don't want to be transported to emotional territories where they don't know how to react. **Hector Babenko**

Money Mastery

All riches have their origin in mind. Wealth is in ideas - not money. **Robert Collier**

Day # 21

Fitness Facts

The more physical activity you engage in, the more time you should devote to flexibility & stretching work.

Spiritual Quotes

The will is a product of integrity, not a child of contradictions. **N. Sri Ram**

Quote of the Day

One hundred percent of the shots you don't take don't go in. **Wayne Gretzky**

Food Facts

Rice paper does not contain one grain of rice - it's made from either Rice straw, Bamboo, Hemp, Mulberry leaves, Wingceltis, or Gampi.

Mind Massage

In Mr. Powell's family, there are one grandfather, one grandmother, two fathers, two mothers, one father-in-law, one mother-in-law, four children, three grandchildren, one brother, two sisters, two sons, two daughters, and one daughter-in-law.

How many members are there in Mr. Powell's family? Give minimal possible answer.

Emotion

I-can't-stand-it: imagining one can't tolerate situations or have any happiness if the situation persists. **John W. Maag**

Money Mastery

A simple fact that is hard to learn is that the time to save money is when you have some. **Joe Moore**

Day # 22

Fitness Facts

Exercise helps elevate your mood and keeps depression at bay.

Spiritual Quotes

Three things in human life are important. The first is to be kind. The second is to be kind. And the third is to be kind. **Henry James**

Quote of the Day

The battles that count aren't the ones for gold medals. The struggles within yourself - the invisible, inevitable battles inside all of us - that's where it's at. **Jesse Owens**

Food Facts

Vegemite is an Australian icon, which was developed in 1922 by Dr. Cyril Callister. He took used brewer's yeast and blended the yeast extract with ingredients like celery, onion, salt, and a few secret ingredients to make this paste rich in B vitamins; it was developed for the Fred Walker Company, which is now Kraft Foods.

Mind Massage

When Alexander the Great attacked the forces of Porus, the Greeks captured an Indian soldier. He had displayed such bravery in battle, however, that the enemy offered to let him choose how he wanted to be killed. They told him, "If you tell a lie, you will be put to the sword, and if you tell the truth you will be hanged." The soldier could make only one statement. He made that statement and went free. What did he say?

Emotion

Think about any attachments that are depleting your emotional reserves. Consider letting them go. **Oprah Winfrey**

Money Mastery

It is more rewarding to watch money change the world than watch it accumulate. **Gloria Steinem**

Day # 23

Fitness Facts

Lifestyle physical activity, such as taking the stairs, gardening, and walking instead of driving, is as effective as structured gym workouts in improving fitness.

Spiritual Quotes

If you judge people, you have no time to love them. **Mother Teresa**

Quote of the Day

Nothing will ever be attempted if all possible objections must be overcome first. **Anonymous**

Food Facts

Ten gallon hats only hold about 6 pints or 2.8 Litres.

Mind Massage

What is round as a dishpan, deep as a tub, and still the oceans couldn't fill it up?

Emotion

By taking control of our emotions and minimizing the degree to which we indulge in negative emotions (and all negative emotions are basically a form of self-indulgence), we not only increase our personal freedom, but we also become vastly more effective and efficient human beings.

Money Mastery

An important lever for sustained action in tackling poverty and reducing hunger is money. **Gro Harlem Brundtland**

Day # 24

Fitness Facts

Improving fitness appears to help men live longer following a heart attack.

Spiritual Quote

Believe nothing, no matter where you read it, or who said it, no matter if I have said it, unless it agrees with your own reason and your own common sense. **Buddha**

Quote of the Day

Courage is going from failure to failure without losing enthusiasm. **Winston Churchill**

Food Facts

Tea strengthens bones because isoflavonoid chemicals in tea may have a weak estrogenic effect, reducing bone deterioration and osteoporosis risk.

Mind Massage

A state has a law stating that no man or woman can marry more than once within that state. There is a man that legally marries more than 10 times in that same state. Who is that man?

Emotion

My house is my refuge, an emotional piece of architecture, not a cold piece of convenience. **Luis Barragan**

Money Mastery

A fool and his money are soon parted. **Thomas Tusser**

Day # 25

Fitness Facts

When you improve your strength and stamina, it's easier to accomplish everyday tasks like carrying the groceries and climbing the stairs.

Spiritual Quote

Happiness cannot be traveled to, owned, earned, worn or consumed. Happiness is the spiritual experience of living every minute with love, grace and gratitude. **Denis Waitley**

Quote of the Day

If we are to have real peace, we must begin with the children. **Mahatma Gandhi**

Food Facts

Olive oil has lots of anti-oxidants and anti-inflammatory properties to fight rheumatoid arthritis.

Mind Massage

There is a two-digit number, the second digit of which is 4 less than its first digit. Also, the number is divisible by the sum of its digits and if you do so, the quotient would be 7. Find the number.

Emotion

Condemning and damning - the tendency to be excessively critical of oneself, others, or the world. **John W. Maag**

Money Mastery

Wealth flows from energy and ideas. **William Feather**

Day # 26

Fitness Facts

Some exercise is better than none and even small amounts of activity will have a positive effect on weight control.

Spiritual Quote

Blessed are the meek, for they shall inherit the earth. **Jesus of Nazareth**

Quote of the Day

Bureaucracy defends the status quo long past the time when the quo has lost its status. **Laurence J. Peter**

Food Facts

Mel Blanc (voice of Bugs Bunny) was allergic to carrots.

Mind Massage

Because cigars cannot be entirely smoked, a hobo who collects cigar butts can make a cigar to smoke out of every 3 butts that he finds. Today, he has collected 27 cigar butts. How many cigars will he be able to smoke?

Emotion

An effective way to pull yourself out of an emotional slump, like a mild depression, is to describe your emotional state out loud or in writing. When you do this exercise, try to describe yourself as if you were another person.

Money Mastery

All my life I knew that there was all the money you could want out there. All you have to do is go after it. **Curtis Carlson**

Day # 27

Fitness Facts

Exercise increases energy levels and reduces stress, which can improve your life as well as the lives of everyone else around you.

Spiritual Quote

Not a shred of evidence exists in favour of the idea that life is serious. **Brendan Gill**

Quote of the Day

The true measure of a man is how he treats someone who can do him absolutely no good. **Ann Landers**

Food Facts

Eggs contain most of the recognized vitamins with the exception of vitamin C.

Mind Massage

Decipher the following:
YYRUYYUBICURYY4ME

Emotion

Children who cling to parents or who don't want to leave home are stunted in their emotional, psychological growth. **Dirk Benedict**

Money Mastery

My goal wasn't to make a ton of money. It was to build good computers. **Steve Wozniak**

Day # 28

Fitness Facts

The length of time we live may be relatively fixed, but the quality of that time is totally within your control. By exerting some control over your well-being with exercise and moderate diet, the life you lead can become much more pleasant and healthy.

Spiritual Quote

Can one behave the same inwardly, whatever the circumstances? Can one's behaviour spring from within and not depend on what people think of you or how they look at you? **Jiddu Krishnamurti**

Quote of the Day

Peace cannot be kept by force. It can only be achieved by understanding. **Albert Einstein**

Food Facts

Honey is the only food that humans eat that will never go bad.

Mind Massage

Someone at a party introduces you to your mother's only sister's husband's only sister-in-law. She has no brothers.
What do you call this lady?

Emotion

Rose Wilder Lane defined freedom as self-control. Freedom is essentially a matter of achieving more and more control over one's own self.

Money Mastery

Many folks think they aren't good at earning money, when what they don't know is how to use it. **Frank A. Clark**

Day # 29

Fitness Facts

Regular exercise among 60 and 70 year olds can improve their fitness levels to those that are normally associated with men and women that are much younger.

Spiritual Quote

We can never obtain peace in the world if we neglect the inner world and don't make peace with ourselves. World peace must develop out of inner peace. Without inner peace it is impossible to achieve world peace, external peace. Weapons themselves do not act. They have not come out of the blue. Man has made them. But even given those weapons, those terrible weapons, they cannot act by themselves. As long as they are left alone in storage they cannot do any harm. A human being must use them. Someone must push the button. Satan, the evil powers, cannot push that button. Human beings must do it. **The Dalai Lama**

Quote of the Day

Many of us spend half of our time wishing for things we could have, if we didn't spend half of our time wishing. **Anonymous**

Food Facts

In 1900 when Louis Lassen ground beef, broiled it, and served it between two pieces of toast, he had invented the hamburger.

Mind Massage

On one side of a card is written:
"THE SENTENCE ON THE OTHERSIDE OF THIS CARD IS TRUE."
On turning the card over you find:
"THE SENTENCE ON THE OTHERSIDE OF THIS CARD IS FALSE."
Which sentence is true?

Emotion

In the book *Dictionary of Typical Command Phrases*, Richard W. Wetherill states that when we are emotionally upset, we program our brains with faulty and self-destructive programming. When we are in a state of emotional upset we tend to say things such as, "If she does that again, I'll show her!" Or, "I'll never be any good at anything!" These sentences become "command phrases" which are planted in our unconscious mind where they continue to have a powerful destructive affect over us even when our emotions have calmed down.

Money Mastery

Do what you love and the money will follow. **Marsha Sinetar**

Day # 30

Fitness Facts

Most people are sexual throughout their lives, with or without a partner, and some feel greater sexual freedom in their later years. On the other hand, some men and women are content to be sexually inactive.

Spiritual Quote

If you scatter thorns, don't go barefoot. **Italian Proverb**

Quote of the Day

You gain strength, courage, and confidence by every experience in which you really stop to look fear in the face. You must do the thing, which you think you cannot do. **Eleanor Roosevelt**

Food Facts

Chewing gum may keep you slim by boosting the metabolic rate by about 20%.

Mind Massage

How many squares are there in a 5-inch by 5-inch square grid? Note that the grid is made up of one inch by one-inch squares.

Emotion

When we identify ourselves with something – no matter what it is – we are unable to step back and view it objectively. Humans can identify themselves with just about anything, including their emotions. I should say: especially their emotions. Now, when we identify with our emotions, it is very difficult to control them; when we are immersed in our emotions, we are controlled by them. The secret of emotional control is to disengage yourself from them, to pull back, and cease identifying with your feelings and moods.

Money Mastery

I am fiercely loyal to those willing to put their money where my mouth is.
Paul Harvey

Day # 31

Fitness Facts

There are two indicators of age chronological age and physiological age. Chronological age is the number of years that you have lived. Physiological age reflects your biological age and tells how old your body is in respect to your health and disease status.

Spiritual Quote

The highest good is like water.
Water gives life to the ten thousand things and does not strive.
It flows in places men reject and so is like the Tao.
In dwelling, be close to the land.
In meditation, go deep in the heart.
In dealing with others, be gentle and kind.
In speech, be true.
In ruling, be just.
In business, be competent.
In action, watch the timing.
Tao Te Ching

Quote of the Day

Knowledge is proud that she knows so much; Wisdom is humble that she knows no more. **Cowper**

Food Facts

Cherries are a member of the rose family.
Mind Massages
A blue house has blue bricks.
 A red house has red bricks.
A yellow house has yellow bricks.
A orange house has orange bricks.
What color bricks does a green house have?

Emotion

Security represents your sense of worth, your identity, your emotional anchorage, your self-esteem, your basic personal strength or lack of it. **Stephen R. Covey**

Money Mastery

If the money we donate helps one child or can ease the pain of one parent, those funds are well spent. **Carl Karcher**

Day # 32

Fitness Facts

The key to a healthy, happy life style is to be patient. Rome wasn't built in a day nor will you.

Spiritual Quote

Zen mind is not Zen mind. That is, if you are attached to Zen mind, then you have a problem, and your way is very narrow. Throwing away Zen mind is correct Zen mind. Only keep the question, "What is the best way of helping other people?" **Seung Sahn**

Quote of the Day

No amount of ability is of the slightest avail without honour. **Andrew Carnegie**

Food Facts

Chicken is one of the few things that we eat before it's born and after it's dead.

Mind Massages

Two people enter a race in which you run to a point and back. Person A runs 20 mph to and from the point. Person B runs to the point going 10 mph and 30 mph going back. Who came in first?

Emotion

Vivid images are like a beautiful melody that speaks to you on an emotional level. It bypasses your logic centres and even your intellect and goes to a different part of the brain. **Steven Bochco**

Money Mastery

Let us not be satisfied with just giving money. Money is not enough, money can be got, but they need your hearts to love them. So, spread your love everywhere you go. **Mother Teresa**

Day # 33

Fitness Facts

It takes 3500 Calories to make a pound of fat! So, as long as you don't overeat, the calories you do eat don't have too much of a chance to turn into fat.

Spiritual Quote

Teach this triple truth to all: A generous heart, kind speech, and a life of service and compassion are the things, which renew humanity. **Buddha**

Quote of the Day

To go against the dominant thinking of your friends, of most of the people you see every day, is perhaps the most difficult act of heroism you can perform. **Theodore H. White**

Food Facts

Cranberries are sorted for ripeness by bouncing them; a fully ripened cranberry will bounce like a basketball.

Mind Massages

An old tea merchant in New York's Chinatown was trying to figure out how to divide 20 pounds of tea into 2-pound packets using a simple balance scale. But this merchant could only find two weights around the shop - one was 5 pounds and the other was 9 pounds.

Can you figure out how he did it?

Emotion

Learning how to monitor your automatic thoughts is not difficult. It is simply a matter of turning your attention inward and tracing back the series of thoughts which ran through your head just prior to experiencing the emotion.

Money Mastery

Too many people spend money they haven't earned to buy things they don't want to impress people they don't like. **Will Smith**

Day # 34

Fitness Facts

If you want to keep your metabolism in high gear, add strength training to your aerobic workouts. You'll build calorie-burning muscle while you're working off excess fat.

Spiritual Quote

God doesn't look at how much we do, but with how much love we do it. **Mother Teresa**

Quote of the Day

Our nation is a rainbow - red, yellow, brown, black, and white - and we're all precious in God's sight. **Jesse Jackson**

Food Facts

In 1922 when Stephen Poplawski put a spinning blade at the bottom of a small electric appliance to make Horlick's malted milk shakes, he had invented the blender.

Mind Massage

Three articles - B1, B2 and B3 - were sold from a Shopping Mall. From the information given below can you discover each article's price and date on which it was sold?
The articles were sold on Nov 10, Nov 12, and Nov 14, one on each day
The article prices were $70, $75, and $80
The article B2 was not sold on Nov 10
The article sold on Nov 10 was $10 higher than that of article B3
The article sold on Nov 14 was for $75

Emotion

My emotional and intellectual response to Hiroshima was that the question of the social responsibility of a journalist was posed with greater urgency than ever. **Wilfred Burchett**

Money Mastery

If you don't have integrity, you have nothing. You can't buy it. You can have all the money in the world, but if you are not a moral and ethical person, you really have nothing. **Henry Kravis**

Day # 35

Fitness Facts

If you're having trouble sleeping, you might want to try late afternoon workouts. Try not to exercise too close to bedtime, as it may make you too alert to drift off. A dip in body temperature (a cool shower) a few hours after you exercise may also help you to fall asleep.

Spiritual Quote

A man's true wealth here after is the good he does in this world to his fellow man. **Muhammad**

Quote of the Day

Into the house where joy lives, happiness will gladly come. **Japanese Proverb**

Food Facts

Why do people say that a poor eater "eats like a bird?" Birds eat half their own body weight in food each day!

Mind Massage

49 friends attended a campfire. After shaking hands, each of them sat on the round table and clinked their mug with the friends to his immediate left and immediate right.

How many times did the mugs clink?

Emotion

In the rush and turmoil of life, we often forget to hold onto what is good about our lives. Take a moment now, to think about all you have been given - life, freedom, others to love.

Money Mastery

If money is your hope for independence you will never have it. The only real security that a man will have in this world is a reserve of knowledge, experience, and ability. **Henry Ford**

Day # 36

Fitness Facts

Every minute of your day is precious. When you train enjoy it.

Spiritual Quote

Achievement seems to be connected with action. Successful men and women keep moving. They make mistakes, but they don't quit. **Conrad Hilton**

Quote of the Day

Above all things, never be afraid. The enemy who forces you to retreat is himself afraid of you at that very moment. **Andre Maurois**

Food Facts

Butter and margarine are similar in calories; the difference is that butter is higher in saturated fats, while margarine generally has more unsaturated fats.

Mind Massage

Sam and Mala have a conversation.
Sam says I am certainly not over 40
Mala says I am 38 and you are at least 5 years older than me
Now Sam says you are at least 39
All the statements by the two are false. How old are they really?

Emotion

If you don't like the way you are feeling or acting, simply make changes in the way you think. This is called "cognitive therapy."

Money Mastery

Time is more value than money. You can get more money, but you cannot get more time. **Jim Rohn**

Day # 37

Fitness Facts

If you have been sedentary the key is to get in shape gradually. A tough workout will make you feel fatigued, sore, and stiff and may even increase the risk of a sudden heart attack.

Spiritual Quote

Every person, all the events of your life, are there because you have drawn them there. What you choose to do with them is up to you. **Richard Bach**

Quote of the Day

In the province of the mind, what one believes to be true either is true or becomes true. **John Lilly**

Food Facts

Casein, the main protein found in milk is the best-known neutralizer for Capsaicin, which makes hot peppers "hot" to the human mouth.

Mind Massage

What is put on a table, cut, but never eaten?

Emotion

The emotional, sexual, and psychological stereotyping of females begins when the doctor says: It's a girl. **Shirley Chisholm**

Money Mastery

Money and success don't change people; they merely amplify what is already there. **Will Smith**

Day # 38

Fitness Facts

It takes about 12 weeks to see measurable changes in your body once you have started an exercise program. However, you will likely notice an increase in your strength and endurance after a few weeks.

Spiritual Quote

Let your courage mount with difficulties. There would be no will if there were no resistance. **N. Sri Ram**

Quote of the Day

Be as careful of the books you read, as of the company you keep; for your habits and character will be as much influenced by the former as by the latter. **Paxton Hood**

Food Facts

Celery requires more calories to eat and digest than it contains.

Mind Massage

What goes up the chimney down, but can't go down the chimney up?

Emotion

Pessimism is essentially a bad habit or bad programming that was developed from being exposed to poor examples from parents, teachers, or others who provided major influences during the formative years of our lives.

Money Mastery

I think the person who takes a job in order to live - that is to say, for the money - has turned himself into a slave. **Joseph Campbell**

Day # 39

Fitness Facts

Sweat is not an indicator of weight loss. The water you lose you will gain back when you drink after your workout.

Spiritual Quote

True understanding is possible only when we are fully conscious of our thought, not as an operative observer on this thought, but completely and without the intervention of a choice.
Jiddu Krishnamurti

Quote of the Day

The real voyage of discovery consists not in seeking new landscapes but in having new eyes. **Marcel Proust**

Food Facts

Avocado has the highest protein and oil content of all fruits. The oil, however, is of the healthier unsaturated type.

Mind Massage

There are 4 mugs placed upturned on the table. Each mug has the same number of marbles and a statement about the number of marbles in it. The statements are: Two or Three, One or Four, Three or One, One or Two. Only one of the statements is correct. How many marbles are there under each mug?

Emotion

A man's moral worth is not measured by what his religious beliefs are but rather by what emotional impulses he has received from Nature during his lifetime. **Albert Einstein**

Money Mastery

I never attempt to make money on the stock market. I buy on the assumption that they could close the market the next day and not reopen it for five years. **Warren Buffett**

Day # 40

Fitness Facts

Women with heart disease or arthritis actually experience improved daily function from involvement in various modes of physical activity.

Spiritual Quote

Loneliness and the feeling of being unwanted is the most terrible poverty. **Mother Teresa**

Quote of the Day

Creativity can solve almost any problem. The creative act, the defeat of habit by originality, overcomes everything. **George Lois**

Food Facts

It has been a tradition to serve fish with a slice of lemon since the Middle Ages, when people believed that lemon juice would dissolve any bones accidentally swallowed.

Mind Massage

It happens once in a minute, twice in a week, and once in a year? What is it?

Emotion

That deep emotional conviction of the presence of a superior reasoning power, which is revealed in the incomprehensible universe, forms my idea of God. **Albert Einstein**

Money Mastery

Money won't create success, the freedom to make it will. **Nelson Mandela**

Day # 41

Fitness Facts

The saying "No pain, no gain." is not true. Exercise doesn't need to hurt. Muscle soreness when you do something new isn't unusual, but soreness isn't the same as pain.

Spiritual Quote

Our primary purpose in this life is to help others. If you can't help, then at least don't hurt. **The Dalai Lama**

Quote of the Day

Ever tried? Ever failed? No Matter, try again, fail again, Fail better. **Samuel Beckett**

Food Facts

It takes about 10 pounds of milk to make one pound of cheese.

Mind Massage

A boy found that he had a 48-inch strip of paper. He could cut an inch off every second. How long would it take for him to cut 48 pieces? He cannot fold the strip and also cannot stack two or more strips and cut them together.

Emotion

To be a human being means to possess a feeling of inferiority which constantly presses towards its own conquest. The greater the feeling of inferiority that has been experienced,the more powerful is the urge for conquest and the more violent the emotional agitation. **Alfred Adler**

Money Mastery

When I chased after money, I never had enough. When I got my life on purpose and focused on giving of myself and everything that arrived into my life, then I was prosperous. **Wayne Dyer**

Day # 42

Fitness Facts

Studies have suggested that walking at a brisk pace for three or more hours a week can reduce your risk for coronary heart disease by 65 percent.

Spiritual Quote

The love of one's country is a splendid thing. But why should love stop at the border? **Pablo Casals**

Quote of the Day

Comedy is nothing more than tragedy deferred. **Pico Iyer**

Food Facts

Bakers used to be fined if their loaves were under weight, so they used to add an extra loaf to every dozen, in case they were under weight - hence, the expression "baker's dozen."

Mind Massage

Jack and Jill are playing cards for a stake of $1 a game. At the end of the evening, Jack has won 3 games and Jill has won $3. How many games did they play?

Emotion

An important aspect of emotional control is the ability to handle emotional contagion. We can become "infected" by the emotions and moods of others. You can catch both negative and positive emotions alike, such as euphoria, elation, sadness, depression, anger, grief, etc. It is important to develop some steps for protecting yourself from the negative emotions of others. Pay attention to how you feel around different people. Become aware of and label your emotional responses. Examine your emotional responses. Recognizing that a negative emotion actually belongs to someone else, may not be enough to prevent the mood from spreading to you. Never allow yourself to become contaminated with other people's negativity.

Money Mastery

I don't want to make money; I want to make a difference. **Lady Gaga**

Day # 43

Fitness Facts

Walking at a brisk pace (at 15-minute or 4 mph mile) burns nearly as many calories as jogging over the same distance. Jogging takes less time to cover the same distance and benefits the bones; however, it may be too strenuous for some. Train, don't strain.

Spiritual Quotes

The cave you fear to enter holds the treasure you seek. **Joseph Campbell**

Quote of the Day

The wisest men follow their own direction. **Euripides**

Food Facts

When a source of Vitamin C (orange, lemon, grapefruit, strawberry, tomato, potato, etc.) is eaten with meat or cooked dry beans, the body makes better use of the iron in the protein food.

Mind Massage

Bill is at a family reunion. Uncle John tells Bill that Bill has one long lost sister, who always speaks the truth. He points at a table, where three women are sitting and says, "One of those ladies is your long lost sister. Go meet her." Bill goes over to the table as told. "I am your long lost sister," says Sharon. "She's lying, I am your long lost sister," says Barbara with a smirk. Julia looks at Bill and says, "Two of us always lie."
Which one is Bill's long lost sister?

Emotion

Painful as it may be, a significant emotional event can be the catalyst for choosing a direction that serves us - and those around us - more effectively. Look for the learning. **Louisa May Alcott**

Money Mastery

No one would remember the Good Samaritan if he'd only had good intentions; he had money as well. **Margaret Thatcher**

Day # 44

Fitness Facts

For complete fitness you need to include aerobic exercise, strength training, and stretching.

Spiritual Quote

Life is both pleasure and pain, is it not? ... But why should we cling to pleasure and avoid pain? Why not merely live with both? ... If you cling to pleasure what happens? You get attached, do you not? **Jiddu Krishnamurti**

Quote of the Day

I used to dread getting older because I thought I would not be able to do all the things I wanted to do, but now that I am older I find that I don't want to do them. **Nancy Astor**

Food Facts

The dish Chop-Suey was created by Chinese immigrants in California.

Mind Massage

A farmer built a fence around his 25 cows in a square region. He built it in such a way that one could see 5 poles from any of the four sides.
What is the minimum number of poles the farmer must have used?

Emotion

Emotional occasions, especially violent ones, are extremely potent in precipitating mental rearrangements. The sudden and explosive ways in which love, jealousy, guilt, fear, remorse, or anger can seize upon one are known to everybody.... And emotions that come in this explosive way seldom leave things as they found them. **William James**

Money Mastery

If you don't want to work you have to work to earn enough money so that you won't have to work. **Ogden Nash**

Day # 45

Fitness Facts

If you aren't already Mr. Universe or Ms. America chances are you won't be now, so set reasonable fitness goals so that they can be reasonably attained.

Spiritual Quote

A student asked Soen Nakagawa during a meditation retreat, "I am very discouraged. What should I do?" Soen replied, "Encourage others." **Soen Nakagawa**

Quote of the Day

Work is not always required... there is such a thing as sacred idleness, the cultivation of which is now fearfully neglected. **George McDonald**

Food Facts

The longer that fruits or vegetables sit around, the more nutrients they lose. But fruits and vegetables grown for freezing are usually frozen right away and, therefore, have less time to lose their nutrients.

Mind Massage

An anthropologist discovers an isolated tribe whose written alphabet contains only six letters (call the letters A, B, C, D, E and F). The tribe has a taboo against using the same letter twice in the same word. It's never done.
 If each different sequence of letters constitutes a different word in the language, what is the maximum number of six-letter words that the language can employ?

Emotion

In *The Path of Least Resistance*, Robert Fritz states that most people believe circumstances are the driving force of their lives. In other words, he states that people believe that they are forced to either respond to or react against their circumstances and that they tend not to believe that they can make choices independent of their circumstances.

Money Mastery

An athlete cannot run with money in his pockets. He must run with hope in his heart and dreams in his head. **Emil Zatopek**

Day # 46

Fitness Facts

Exercise may make you feel tired at first, but the tiredness won't last long.

Spiritual Quote

Whatever you have in your mind - forget it; whatever you have in your hand - give it; whatever is to be your fate - face it! **Abu Sa'id**

Quote of the Day

You always pass failure on the way to success. **Mickey Rooney**

Food Facts

Half of the world's population live on a staple diet of rice.

Mind Massage

If you were to dial any 7 digits on a telephone in random order, what is the probability that you will dial your own phone number?
Assume that your telephone number is 7-digits.

Emotion

The worst drugs are as bad as anybody's told you. It's just a dumb trip, which I can't condemn people if they get into it, because one gets into it for one's own personal, social, emotional reasons. It's something to be avoided if one can help it. **John Lennon**

Money Mastery

Money – I make it – I spend it – now it's time to reprogram my thinking and learn from the masters how to save some of it so that it generates enough passive income that will allow me to do what I deem most important in life – physically participating in helping others to find their true potential! **Frank Moffatt**

Day # 47

Fitness Facts

When you exercise wear clothing that is comfortable and allows you to move freely. Also make sure your clothes are cool enough for when your body begins to heat up.

Spiritual Quote

The secret of attraction is to love yourself. Attractive people judge neither themselves nor others. They are open to gestures of love. They think about love, and express their love in every action. They know that love is not a mere sentiment, but the ultimate truth at the heart of the universe. **Deepak Chopra**

Quote of the Day

If you really do put a small value on upon yourself, rest assured that the rest of the world will not raise your price. **Anonymous**

Food Facts

A low calorie diet won't help you lose weight. Low calorie diets may appear at first to help, but soon all weight loss comes to a halt when your metabolism shuts down. The key is to eat 6 **"small"** meals a day and keep the fat burning engines at full speed. Don't starve yourself.

Mind Massage

I have four wings, but cannot fly
I never laugh and never cry
on the same spot I'm always found,
toiling away with little sound.
What am I?

Emotion

Start by remembering what is important. Most of what stresses us are the things that don't matter in the long run. Being cut off in traffic, breaking a fingernail, not being able to buy the newest gadget, someone else's rudeness – these are not worth worrying about. What really matters is whether we are fair and caring.

Money Mastery

Money was never a big motivation for me, except as a way to keep score. The real excitement is playing the game. **Donald Trump**

Day # 48

Fitness Facts

Proper footwear should be comfortable by providing adequate arch support and sole protection.

Spiritual Quote

If you don't get what you want, you suffer; if you get what you don't want, you suffer; even when you get exactly what you want, you still suffer because you can't hold on to it forever. Your mind is your predicament. It wants to be free of change. Free of pain, free of the obligations of life and death. But change is a law, and no amount of pretending will alter that reality. **Dan Millman**

Quote of the Day

Focus + Determination + Hard Work = Talent **Frank Moffatt**

Food Facts

The only vegetable or fruit which is never sold frozen, canned, processed or cooked is lettuce. Lettuce is only sold fresh.

Mind Massage

As I was traveling to Calgary I saw a man with 7 wives, with 7 kittens, in 7 sacks, and with 7 drinks on a bike.
How many people/things are going to Calgary?

Emotion

In order to experience emotion we need to first interpret an event or stimulus and assign meaning to it. Although we may not have control over the event, we can learn how to control our interpretation process, thus increasing our emotional control.

Money Mastery

A rich man is nothing but a poor man with money. **W. C. Fields**

Day # 49

Fitness Facts

Today there are many options when one decides, where, when and with whom to workout. Remember, the choice is yours if you aren't happy, change it.

Spiritual Quote

You yourself, as much as anybody in the entire universe, deserve your love and affection. **Buddha**

Quote of the Day

A non-doer is very often a critic - that is, someone who sits back and watches doers, and then waxes philosophically about how the doers are doing. It's easy to be a critic, but being a doer requires effort, risk, and change. **Dr. Wayne Dyer**

Food Facts

Shredded wheat was the first breakfast cereal to ever be produced.

Mind Massage

Which candle burns longer a blue candle or a green candle?

Emotion

The quality of your life is dependent upon the quality of the life of your cells. If the bloodstream is filled with waste products, the resulting environment does not promote a strong, vibrant, healthy cell life - nor a biochemistry capable of creating a balanced emotional life for an individual. **Anthony Robbins**

Money Mastery

God wants us to prosper financially, to have plenty of money, to fulfill the destiny He has laid out for us. **Joel Osteen**

Day # 50

Fitness Facts

An exercise program can be a fun addition to your week that doesn't have to cramp your schedule. Do a variety of exercises, set realistic goals, and enjoy yourself.

Spiritual Quote

The great awareness comes slowly, piece by piece. The path of spiritual growth is a path of lifelong learning. The experience of spiritual power is basically a joyful one. **Scott Peck**

Quote of the Day

Don't be pushed by your problems. Be led by your dreams. **Anonymous**

Food Facts

Refried beans aren't really what they seem. Although their name seems like a reasonable translation of Spanish frijoles refritos, the fact is the beans aren't fried twice. In Spanish, refritos literally means "well-fried" not "re-fried."

Mind Massage

Only one color, but not one size
Stuck at the bottom, but easily flies
Present in the sun, but not in the rain
Doing no harm, and feeling no pain
What am I?

Emotional

Scientific knowledge and the wisdom of the ages agree the healthiest people live lives based on trying to make the world a better place for all living creatures. You cannot be emotionally fit if your heart is full of anger or hate.

Money Mastery

Successful people make money. It's not that people who make money become successful, but that successful people attract money. They bring success to what they do. **Wayne Dyer**

Fifty

Fitness Exercises

Cardio Exercises

There are many variations of cardio exercises. We have listed 4 here but please feel free to do whatever works best for you. There are no descriptions for these exercises as they are self explanatory.

- Tread Mill (Walking or Jogging)
- Elliptical
- Exercise Bike
- Stairmaster or Stair Climber

Neck Exercises

Manual Neck Resistance - Place the heel of your hand on your forehead. Apply pressure with your hand. Resist against this pressure with your neck muscles. Press as hard as you can, but don't over do it and run the risk of an injury.

Neck Stretch - Turn your head as far as you can so your chin is over, or close to over, your shoulder, and then hold for 20 seconds. Repeat the stretch on the other side. Don't hold your breath.

Shoulder Exercises

Military Press – Sitting on a bench, grab the barbell with a wider than shoulder width grip. Push the barbell directly upward until it is at arms length above your shoulders. Lower the barbell back to starting position. Repeat for 8 to 12 repetitions.

Seated Dumbbell Press - Sit on an upright bench. Lift two dumbbells to your shoulders. Your palms should be facing forwards. Push the dumbbells directly upward until your arms are straight but not locked out. Lower the dumbbells back to the starting position at the top of your chest. Repeat for 8 to 12 repetitions.

Side Lateral Raises - Stand with your feet shoulder width apart. Hold the dumbbells in front of your body with your palms facing each other. Keep your elbows bent at approximately 90-degrees. Raise the dumbbells out to the sides and upwards to shoulder level. Hold this position for a second to maximize the contraction. Lower the dumbbells back to the starting position. Repeat for 8 to 12 repetitions.

Front Lateral Raises - Stand with your feet shoulder width apart. Hold the dumbbells in front of your body with your palms facing in towards your legs. Slightly bend your elbows. Raise the dumbbells to the front and upwards to shoulder level. Hold this position for a second to maximize the contraction. Lower the dumbbells back to the starting position. Repeat for 8 to 12 repetitions.

Bent Lateral Raises - Bend over at the waist with your knees slightly bent and your feet shoulder width apart. Hold the dumbbells at arms length in front of you with your palms facing each other and your elbows slightly bent. Raise the dumbbells to the back and upwards as far as possible. Hold this position for a second to maximize the contraction. Lower the dumbbells back to the starting position. Repeat for 8 to 12 repetitions.

Barbell Shrugs - Bend your legs and lift the barbell until it is at arms length in front of you. Keep your knees slightly bent to take the stress off of your lower back. Without moving your arms, lift the barbell upwards with your shoulders as high as you can. Hold this position for a second at the top of the movement to maximize the contraction. Lower the barbell back to the starting position. Repeat for 8 to 12 repetitions.

Shoulder Stretch - This stretch will mainly affect the front of the shoulder (the deltoid muscle). Place one arm across the front of your body. With the opposite hand, grasp your elbow. Now, pull your arm across your body without twisting your torso.

Arm Exercises – Biceps

Standing Barbell Curls – Hold the barbell with an underhand grip. Stand with your feet shoulder width apart. Let the barbell hang in front of you at arms length. Keep your elbows close to your side at all times. Use your biceps to curl the barbell up to shoulder level. Hold the weight in the top position for a second to maximize the contraction of your biceps. Now slowly lower the barbell to the starting position.

Repeat for 8 to 12 repetitions.

Standing Dumbbell Curls - Hold the dumbbells with an underhand grip. Stand with your feet shoulder width apart. Let the dumbbells hang at arms length on each side of your body. Keep your elbows close to your sides at all times. Use your biceps to curl the dumbbells up to shoulder level. Hold the weight in the top position for a second to maximize the contraction of your biceps. Now slowly lower the dumbbells to the starting position. Repeat for 8 to 12 repetitions.

Dumbbell Concentration Curls - Sit legs apart at the end of an exercise bench. Brace your elbow against the inside of your knee and fully straighten your arm. Use your bicep to curl the dumbbell up to shoulder level. Hold the weight in the top position for a second or two to maximize the contraction of your biceps. Now slowly lower the dumbbell to the starting position. Repeat for 8 to 12 repetitions. Do the same for each arm.

Bicep-Wall Stretch - Place the palm, inner elbow, and shoulder of one arm against the wall. Keeping the arm in contact with the wall, exhale and slowly turn your body around, to feel the stretch in your biceps and chest.

Arm Exercises – Triceps

Lying Barbell Extensions - Lie on your back on a flat bench. Your feet should be shoulder width apart on each side of the bench. It is best to have a training partner hand you the barbell. Hold the bar narrower than shoulder width. Press the barbell up until it is at arms length above your shoulders. Lower the barbell to within an inch or so above your forehead. Using your triceps push the bar back up to the starting position. Repeat for 8 to 12 repetitions.

Tricep Dumbbell Extensions - Stand with your feet shoulder width apart. Lift the dumbbell so that it is straight above your shoulder. Slightly bend your knees to take the pressure off of your lower back. Slowly lower the dumbbell to a position behind your head and where your elbow is at a 90-degree angle. Slowly lift the dumbbell back to the starting position. Repeat for 8 to 12 repetitions. Do the same for each arm.

Tricep Pushdowns - Attach a short bar or rope apparatus to an overhead pulley. Stand with your feet shoulder width apart. Grab the bar or rope with an overhand grip. Hold your arms at a 90-degree to your body and keep your elbows against your sides at all times during the exercise. Push the bar down until your arms are straight. Hold this position for a second to maximize the contraction. Slowly lower the weight until the arms are again at 90-degrees. Repeat for 8 to 12 repetitions.

Tricep Dumbbell Kick Backs - Stand beside a flat exercise bench. Bend over until your upper body is parallel to the floor. Place one hand on the bench to support yourself. Hold the weight at a 90-degree angle to your upper body. Lift the dumbbell until your arm is straight. Hold this position for a second or two to maximize the contraction in the triceps. Slowly return the dumbbell to the starting position. Repeat for 8 to 12 repetitions.

Tricep Stretch

Hold one end of a towel in your right hand. Raise and bend your right arm to drape the towel down your back. Keep your right arm in this position and continue holding onto the towel. Reach behind your lower back and grasp the bottom end of the towel with your left hand. Climb your left hand progressively higher up the towel, which also pulls your right arm down. Continue until your hands touch, or as close as you can comfortably go. Switch arms and repeat.

Forearm Exercise

Reverse Curls – Hold a barbell palms down and shoulder width apart. Stand with your feet shoulder width apart. Let the barbell hang in front of you. Keep your elbows close to your sides at all times. Curl the barbell up to shoulder level. Hold this position for a second to maximize the contraction. Slowly lower the barbell to the starting position. Repeat for 8 to 12 repetitions.

Wrist Exercises

Wrist Curl Rolls – At one end of a 6 or 7 foot piece of rope tie a 5 or 10 lb weight. At the other end of the rope tie a dumbbell bar or twelve inch piece of wood dowel. Hold the end with the dumbbell bar at shoulder height, arms extended, palms down. Begin rolling up the rope by first twisting your right wrist forward and then by twisting your left wrist forward. Continue until you have rolled the weight up to the bar. Now reverse the action until the weight has been rolled back down to ground level. Repeat 4 times or as many times as possible.

Dumbbell Wrist Curls - Keep the palms of your hands facing up. Sit on a flat exercise bench with your forearms resting on your thighs and your wrists hanging over the ends of your knees. Curl the dumbbells up using only your wrists. Hold the dumbbells at the top position for a second to maximize the contraction. Slowly lower the dumbbells back to the starting position. Repeat for 8 to 12 repetitions.

Wrist Stretch -
Place hands together, in praying position. Slowly raise elbows so arms are parallel to ground, keeping hands flat against each other. Hold position for 10 to 30 seconds.

Chest Exercises

Flat Barbell Bench Press - Lie down on the flat bench press. Place your feet flat on the floor or on the end of the bench. Hold the bar with a wider than shoulder width grip. Once you have lifted the bar from the rack, position the bar over your chest. Lower the barbell until your elbows are at 90-degrees to the floor, parallel with the bench. Then press the bar back up to a position just short of locking out your elbows. Repeat for 8 to 12 repetitions. Lowering the bar past 90-degrees may cause serious shoulder injury.

Incline Dumbbell Press - Lower the dumbbells until your elbows are at a 90-degree angle to your shoulders. Then press the dumbbells back up to a position just short of locking out your elbows. Repeat for 8 to 12 repetitions. This exercise would require an incline weight lifting bench to be performed at home. Lowering the dumbbells past 90-degrees may cause serious shoulder injury.

Decline Barbell Bench Press - Lower the barbell until your elbows are at a 90-degree angle to your shoulders. Then press the bar back up to a position just short of locking out your elbows. Repeat for 8 to 12 repetitions. This exercise would require a decline weight lifting bench to be performed at home. Lowering the bar past 90-degrees may cause serious shoulder injury.

Dumbbell Bench Press - Lie down on a flat bench. Lower the dumbbells until your elbows are at a 90-degree angle to the floor, parallel with the bench. Then press the dumbbells back up to a position just short of locking out your elbows. Repeat for 8 to 12 repetitions. Lowering the dumbbells past 90-degrees may cause serious shoulder injury.

Push Ups - Lie face down on the floor with your palms on the ground beside your body. Keeping your legs and torso straight, push yourself up with your arms until they are extended. Lower yourself slowly until your chest nearly touches the floor. Hold this position for a second. Again push yourself back up to where you started. Repeat for 8 to 12 repetitions.

Corner Stretch for Chest - Forget all your grade school fears - standing in a corner is one of the best stretching exercises. Stand facing a corner with one hand on each wall, about chin level. Lean forward until you feel a stretch in your chest and shoulders. Repeat this muscle stretching technique for flexibility.

Back Exercises

One Arm Dumbbell Row – Put one knee on a flat exercise bench and one foot on the floor. For support place one hand on the bench. Hold the dumbbell with your other hand. Keep your back level with the floor. Keeping your elbow close to your side, slowly pull the dumbbell directly upwards until it touches your side. Hold it there for a second to maximize the contraction. Lower the dumbbell slowly, back to the starting position. Repeat for 8 to 12 repetitions. Do the same for both arms.

Bent Over Barbell Row - Bend over and grab a barbell with your hands shoulder width apart. Keep your knees slightly bent. Lift the bar keeping your arms straight. Keep your upper body at a 45-degree angle to the floor. Using just your arms raise the barbell to your stomach. Hold this position for a second to maximize the contraction. Lower the bar until your arms are straight, but don't let the barbell touch the floor. Repeat for 8 to 12 repetitions.

Lat Pulldowns – Hold the bar with your hands slightly wider than shoulder width apart. Pull the bar down in front of your head until the bar nearly touches the top of your chest. Hold this position for a second to maximize the contraction. Slowly straighten your arms back to the starting position. Repeat for 8 to 12 repetitions.

Back Extension Using The Stability Ball - Lie face down on a stability ball. Position yourself so you are balanced directly over the ball with your toes or the sides of your feet on he floor. Lower your upper body towards the ground. Place your hands on your chest and raise your upper body as high as possible. Repeat for 8 to 12 repetitions.

Back Stretch - With this exercise, you release all that tension and stress you're holding in your shoulders and upper back. Kneel with your knees under hips and hands under shoulders. Spread the fingers out on the floor with palms flat and contract the abdominal muscles to bring the head, neck, and back in alignment. Inhale and tip the hip bones towards the ceiling while drawing the shoulders back and down away from your ears and look up. Exhale and tuck the chin while pulling your belly towards your spine. Round the back and feel a stretch down your spine. Repeat for 4 to 6 breaths, moving smoothly between each move.

Abdominal Exercises

Bicycle Manoeuvre - Lie flat on the floor with your lower back against the ground. Put your hands beside your head. Bring your knees up to about a 45-degree angle and slowly go through a bicycle pedal motion. Touch your left elbow to your right knee and then your right elbow to your left knee.

Crunch on an Exercise Ball - Sit on the exercise ball with your feet flat on the floor. Let the ball roll back slowly and lie back until your thighs and torso are parallel with the floor. Contract your abdominals raising your torso to no more than 45 degrees.

Leg Exercises

Leg Press – Place your feet shoulder width apart on the platform. Grasp the handles beside the seat. Push back against the platform. Don't completely straighten the leg to avoid injury. Return to starting position. Repeat for 8 to 12 repetitions.

Box Squats – Standing shoulder width apart, hold the bar wider than shoulder width apart. Position the bar across the top of your shoulders and not on your neck. Lift the bar off of the rack with your legs. Look forward. Bend your legs and squat down. Your knees should be directly over your toes as you do the movement. At the bottom of this squat, sit back on the box and pause for a second before coming up. Repeat for 8 to 12 repetitions.

Lunges - Step out a couple feet with one leg, keep your toes pointed forward and your front foot flat on the floor. Bend your front leg until your knee is at a 90-degree angle to the floor, and your back leg should also bend until it is at a 90-degree angle. Push up and return to the starting position. Repeat for 8 to 12 repetitions, and then do the same with the other leg out front. You can also do lunges with your back leg on a bench; this will give you a better range of motion.

Leg Extensions – Place your feet beneath the roller pads and hold the handles at the sides of the machine. Straighten your legs, lifting the weight. Pause at the top for a second or two to enhance the contraction. Lower your legs slowly to the starting position. Repeat for 8 to 12 repetitions.

Lying Leg Curls - Hook your feet beneath the roller pads and hold the handles at the sides of the machine. Curl your legs, lifting the weight. Pause at the top for a second or two to enhance the contraction. Lower your legs slowly to the starting position. Repeat for 8 to 12 repetitions.

Quad Stretch - For lean sexy legs, do the standing quadriceps stretch. Pull your foot up, with the knee bent and the thigh straight up and down, next to the supporting leg. During this muscle stretching, don´t pull the leg back and to the side, which stresses the knee, and don´t lean forward, which reduces range of motion and decreases stretching effectiveness.

Hamstring Stretch - For a good hamstring stretch, lie on your back on the floor. Leave one leg extended on the floor and raise the other, knee straight, until you feel the stretch in your hamstring. Loop a towel around your leg and hold the ends in your hands to make it easier.

Calf Exercises

Standing Calve Raise - Place your head between the shoulder pads on the calf machine. With your feet shoulder width apart, place the balls of your feet on the foot block, toes pointing forward. Keep your legs straight during the entire movement. Slowly lower your heels until your calve muscles stretch down as far as possible. Hold the stretched position for a second and then rise up as high as you can on your toes. Hold this position for a second to enhance the contraction in the calves. Repeat for 8 to 12 repetitions. This exercise would require a standing calve machine to be performed at home.

Seated Calve Raise - Adjust the kneepads so they are snug and comfortable. With your feet shoulder width apart place the balls of your feet on the foot block, toes pointing forward. Raise your heals up as high as you can. Hold this position for a second to enhance the contraction in the calves. Lower your heels until your calve muscles stretch as far as possible. Hold the stretched position for a second. Repeat for 8 to 12 repetitions. This exercise would require a Standing calve machine to be performed at home.

One Leg Calve Raise - Standing on one leg, place the ball of your foot on a block with your heels hanging over the edge. Hold onto something for balance. Keep your knee straight. Slowly lower your heel until your calf muscle stretches as far as possible. Hold the stretched position for a second and then rise up as high as you can on your toes. Hold this position for a second to enhance the contraction of the calf. Repeat for 8 to 12 repetitions. Repeat with the other leg.

Calf Stretch - Give those calves the muscle stretching of their life! You should stretch your calves two ways with two different stretching exercises. First is the usual way where you lean against a wall, step back with the leg to be stretched, knee straight, then keep your heel down and push your hips forward until you feel the stretching in your calf. Second, keep the same position but bend your knee, which will give a better stretch to the soleus muscle and the achilles´ tendon.

Mind Massage Answers

Methodical Mind Massages – Answers 1 to 50

Answer Q # 1

*A stocking or a sock
*Usually, it is filled with your foot in the morning and taken off (i.e. emptied) at night. But on Christmas, it is emptied at night so that Santa can fill it with gifts. Then it is emptied in the morning by children.

Answer Q # 2

He was Walking. He is a Bus driver. But it does not say that he was driving.

Answer Q # 3

*The next two letters are N and T.
*The pattern is - the last letter of the words onE, twO, threE, fouR, etc...
*Hence, the next two letters are seveN and eighT.

Answer Q # 4

For the sake of explanation, let's identify a 4 gallon bucket as Bucket P and a 9 gallon bucket as Bucket Q.
*Fill bucket Q with 9 gallons of water
*Pour 4 gallons water from bucket Q to bucket P
*Empty bucket P
*Pour 4 gallons water from bucket Q to bucket P
*Empty bucket P
*Pour 1 gallon water from bucket Q to bucket P
*Fill bucket Q with 9 gallons of water
*Pour 3 gallons water from bucket Q to bucket P
*9 gallon bucket now contains 6 gallons of water

Answer Q # 5

* Doc, Happy, Smelly, Sneezy, Stumpy, Sleepy, Grumpy, Dopey, Droopy, Bashful

Answer Q # 6

*Repeat after me.

Answer Q # 7

*There are total 2 couples and so: the grandfather and grandmother, their son and his wife, and their son. So 5 people in total.
*Three - grandfather & grandmother + son & wife + son.

Answer Q # 8

*There are 11 letters in "The Alphabet."

Answer Q # 9

*Darkness, Fog, Smoke.

Answer Q # 10

*The sign-maker will need 192 zeroes.
*Divide 1000 building numbers into groups of 100 each as follow:
(1...100), (101...200), (201...300) ... (901...1000)
*For the first group, the sign-maker will need 11 zeroes.
*For group numbers 2 to 9, he will require 20 zeroes each.
*And for group number 10, he will require 21 zeroes.
*The total numbers of zeroes required are
= 11 + 8*20 + 21 = 11 + 160 + 21 = 192

Answer Q # 11

*It is given that - (sack of potatoes) + (box of mangoes) = (barrel of pickles) + (crate of cherries) and 2 * (crate of cherries) = (box of mangoes)
*Add both the equations
*(sack of potatoes) + (box of mangoes) + 2 * (crate of cherries) = (barrel of pickles) + (crate of cherries) + (box of mangoes)
*(sack of potatoes) + (crate of cherries) = (barrel of pickles)

*(sack of potatoes) + (crate of cherries) = 60 kgs

Answer Q # 12

*It is a one floor house, and a one floor house does not have stairs. Hence, there is no question of colour of stairs as there are no stairs.

Answer Q # 13

*ALL the children are girls, so half are girls and so is the other half.

Answer Q # 14

*There are total 12 members in Mr. Smith's family. Mr. Smith and his wife Debi, nine sons and one daughter.
*Mr. Smith does not have 9 daughters. There is only one daughter and she is the only sister. If there are 9 daughters, then each son will have 9 sisters and not just a one.

Answer Q # 15

*Let distance between home and church be D.
*A person took 4 hours to reach church. So speed while traveling towards church is D/4.
*Similarly, he took 3 hours to reach home. So speed while coming back is D/3.
*There is a speed difference of 7*D/12, which is because the wind is helping the person in one direction and slowing him in the other direction. Average the 2 speeds, and you have the speed that person can travel in no wind, which is 7*D/24.
*Hence, person will take D / (7*D/24) hours to travel distance D which is 24/7 hours.
*Answer is 3 hours 25 minutes 42 seconds

Answer Q # 16

*One of them was a 10 cent coin and the other one was a 50 cent piece.
*The boy got two coins: a 50 cent piece and a 10 cent coin. One of them was not a 50 cent piece. But the other one was.

Answer Q # 17

*It's simple.
*Let's find the possible places horses can finish. Possibilities are:
*Whisper - 2,3,4 (not 5th as Eclipse came one place after him)
*Lightning - 2,3,4
*Eclipse - 3,4,5
*Thunder - 1,3 (not 4th & 5th as Sunshine is two place after him)
*Sunshine - 3,5
*So the result is: 1 Thunder, 2 Lightning, 3 Sunshine, 4 Whisper, 5 Eclipse

Answer Q # 18

*It doesn't matter how you put the marbles in the jar.
*Chances of picking a Red marble are the same. i.e. 50%

Answer Q # 19

*The tape was rewound, which is not possible if it was a suicide.
*The cops knew this was a murder because if it was suicide, the man would be dead and unable to rewind the tape and get it ready for the cops to just push the play button and hear the story.

Answer Q # 20

*The next row is 1113213211
*Starting with the second line, every line describes the line before it. In writing, it is:
One One
Two Ones
One Two One One
etc.

Answer Q # 21

*There are 7 members in Mr. Powell's family. Mother & Father of Mr. Powell, Mr. & Mrs. Powell, his son and two daughters.

*Family Tree - Mother & Father of Mr. Powell + Mr. & Mrs. Powell + one son & two Daughters

Answer Q # 22

*The soldier said, "You will put me to the sword."
*The soldier has to say a Paradox to save himself. If his statement is true, he will be hanged, which is not the sword and hence false. If his statement is false, he will be put to the sword, which will make it true. A Paradox!

Answer Q # 23

*A sieve

Answer Q # 24

*He is a Preacher (Priest) or a Judge, who has the authority to legally marry people.

Answer Q # 25

*Let's assume that the first digit is N. Hence, the second digit is (N-4) and the number is
= 10N + (N-4) = 11N - 4
*Now, it is given that the number is divisible by the sum of its digit and the quotient would be 7.
*(11N - 4) / (N + N - 4) = 7
*(11N - 4) / (2N - 4) = 7
*(11N - 4) = 7 * (2N - 4)
*11N - 4 = 14N - 28
*3N = 24
*N = 8
*Thus, the first digit is 8, the second digit is 4 and the required number is 84.

Answer Q # 26

*He makes 9 originals from the 27 butts he found, and after he

smokes them he has 9 butts left for another 3 cigars. And then he has 3 butts for another cigar.
*So 9+3+1=13

Answer Q # 27

*Too wise are you, too wise you be. I see you are, too wise for me.

Answer Q # 28

*Mother or Mom.

Answer Q # 29

*It's a Paradox. Both the sentences are contradictory to each other. If you say that the first sentence is true, then the second will contradict it and vice versa.

Answer Q # 30

*There are 55 squares in a 5 by 5 grid.
*There are 25 squares of one grid.
*There are 16 squares of four grids i.e. 2 by 2
*There are 9 squares of nine grids i.e. 3 by 3
*There are 4 squares of sixteen grids i.e. 4 by 4
*There is 1 square of twenty-five girds i.e. 5 by 5
*Hence, there are total 25 + 16 + 9 + 4 + 1 = 55 squares.
*You must have noticed that the total number squares possible of each size is always a perfect square i.e. 25, 16, 9, 4, 1

Answer Q # 31

*A green house doesn't have bricks.
*A greenhouse (also called a glasshouse or hothouse) is a building where plants are cultivated.

Answer Q # 32

*Note that initially the speed of Person A (20 mph) was twice the

speed of Person B (10 mph). Hence, when Person A (20 mph forward) reached the point, Person B (10 mph forward) was halfway. When Person A (20 mph back) finished, Person B (still 10 mph forward) reached the point.
*Thus, Person A wins the race and by that time Person B covers only half the distance, no matter how far the point is!!!

Answer Q # 33

*Answer Q # 32 There are many ways to do it.
* Get 4 pounds of tea using 9-pound and 5-pound weights.
* Using the balance, divide this 4 pounds of tea into 2 equal parts of 2 pounds each.
*Using this 2-pound tea packet as a make-shift weight, divide the remaining tea into 9 packets of 2-pounds each.

Answer Q # 34

* B2 was not sold on Nov 10 (clue 3). Neither was it B3 (clue 4). It must have been B1, which was sold on Nov 10, and must have been sold for $80.
* Hence, B3 must have been sold for $70, and B2 must have been sold for $75.
* Also, B2 was sold on Nov 14. It follows that B3 was sold on Nov 12.
* B1 - $80 - Nov 10, B2 - $75 - Nov 14, B3 - $70 - Nov 12

Answer Q # 35

*Let's assume that everyone clinked their mug with a friend to his left only. It means that there are total 49 clinks. Now the right clink of each person is left clink of the person on right which has already happened. Hence, there are only 49 clinks.

Answer Q # 36

* Let's invert the teaser and read it like this :
* Sam says I am certainly over 40
* Mala says I am not 38 and you are at most 4 years older than me

* Now Sam says you are at most 38
* From first the statement it is clear that Sam is over 40. Also, from the next 2 statements it is clear that Mala is less then 38. Hence the possibilities are:
* Sam = 41, 42, 43, 44, 45, ... and Mala = 37, 36, 35, 34, 33, ...
* It also says that the difference between their age is maximum 4 years. Hence, there is only one possible pair i.e. 41 and 37, all other combination are more then 4.
* Hence the answer - Sam is 41 and Mala is 37.

Answer Q # 37

*A deck of cards

Answer Q # 38

*An umbrella

Answer Q # 39

* As it is given that only one of the four statement is correct, the correct number can not appear in more than one statement. If it appears in more than one statement, then more than one statement will be correct.
* Hence, there are 4 marbles under each mug.

Answer Q # 40

* Letter 'e'

Answer Q # 41

*To get 48 pieces, the boy has to put only 47 cuts. i.e. he can cut 46 pieces in 46 seconds. After getting 46 pieces, he will have a 2 inch long piece. He can cut it into two with just a one cut in 1 second. Hence, total of 47 seconds.

Answer Q # 42

* They played a total of 9 games. Jack won 3 games and Jill won 6 games.
* If Jack has won three games and Jill has won $3, she lost a dollar for each loss. Therefore, she has won 6 and lost 3 to make $3, and he won the other 3 that she lost!

Answer Q # 43

* Let's assume that Sharon is Bill's long lost sister. It means that Sharon is telling the truth and Barbara is lying. If so, the statement made by Julia is contradictory. Hence, Sharon is not the sister.
* Barbara is also not the sister, by same reasoning as above.
* Let's assume that Julia is Bill's long lost sister. It means that Julia is telling the truth and other two are lying. Hence, Julia is Bill's long lost sister.

Answer Q # 44

*One pole at each corner and three poles along each side, so that one can always see 5 poles from either of the four sides. The corner pole is shared by two sides, hence reducing the number of poles to 16.

Answer Q # 45

*It is a simple permutation problem of arranging 6 letters to get different six-letter words. And it can be done in 6 ways i.e. 720 ways.
*In other words, the first letter can be any of the given 6 letters (A through F). Then, whatever the first letter is, the second letter will always be from the remaining 5 letters (as same letter cannot be used twice), and the third letter will always be from the remaining 4 letters, and so on. Thus, the different possible six-letter words are $6*5*4*3*2*1 = 720$

Answer Q # 46

*There are 10 digits i.e. 0-9. The first digit can be dialed in 10 ways. The second digit can be dialed in 10 ways. The third digit can be

dialed in 10 ways. And so on.....
*Thus, 7-digit can be dialed in 10*10*10*10*10*10*10 =
(10,000,000) ways. And, you have just one telephone number. Hence,
the possibility that you will dial your own number is 1 in 10,000,000.
*Note that 0123456 may not be a valid 7-digit telephone number.
But while dialing in random order, that is one of the possible 7-digit
numbers which you may dial.

Answer Q # 47

*A windmill. It has four wings but cannot fly. It never laughs or cries.
It is always found on the same spot. And it produces little sound
whenever little wind is there.

Answer Q # 48

*One man is traveling to Calgary. It said, "I saw a man with 7 wives,
with 7 kittens, in 7 sacks, and with 7 drinks, on a bike." He only
saw them, so they did not count. Hence, he is the only person that is
actually going.

Answer Q # 49

*Neither, they both burn shorter. This is a tricky riddle as candles
don't burn longer, they burn shorter. Also, the color of the candles is
just to misguide you.

Answer Q # 50

* A shadow is always Black and comes in different sizes. It is always
stuck at the bottom (i.e. ground) but easily flies. It's always present
in the sun, but not in the rain. And it is doing no harm and feeling no
pain.

Appendix A

(Exercise Program Options)

Please feel free to make up your own program – try to work each body part at least once a week. There is no perfect plan. The only plan that won't work is the one that you don't use. Again, if you are unsure of your current health condition please visit a doctor first prior to starting a workout program.

Routine # 1
Rotate Chest & Shoulders with Arms & Back with Legs and Abs – change exercises daily

Monday
CHEST - Incline Dumbbell Presses
1 set x 15 reps
2-3 sets x 10 reps
SHOULDER TRAINING – Military Press
3-4 x 12-15

Wednesday
BICEPS - Standing Barbell Curls
3 x 15
TRICEPS - Lying Overhead Triceps Extensions
4-6 x 15
FOREARM & WRIST – Reverse curls
3 x 15
BACK MUSCLES - One-Arm Dumbbell Rows
3 sets x 12-15 reps

Friday
LEG MUSCLES - Leg Presses
4-8 x 8-15
Lying Leg Curls
3-6 x 8-10
Seated Calf Raises
3-4 x 12
AB EXERCISES - Crunches
4 x 25

Routine # 2

Rotate Chest, Back, Abs & Shoulders with Arms & Legs – change exercises daily

Monday
CHEST - Incline Dumbbell Presses
1 set x 15 reps
2-3 sets x 10 reps
BACK MUSCLES - One-Arm Dumbbell Rows
3 sets x 12-15 reps
SHOULDER TRAINING – Military Press
3-4 x 12-15
AB EXERCISES - Crunches
4 x 25

Wednesday
BICEPS - Standing Barbell Curls
3 x 15
TRICEPS - Lying Overhead Triceps Extensions
4-6 x 15
FOREARM & WRIST – Reverse curls
3 x 15
LEG MUSCLES - Leg Presses
4-8 x 8-15
Lying Leg Curls
3-6 x 8-10
Seated Calf Raises
3-4 x 12

Friday
CHEST – Flat Barbell Bench Presses
1 set x 15 reps
2-3 sets x 10 reps
BACK MUSCLES – Lat Pulldowns
3 sets x 12-15 reps
SHOULDER TRAINING – Side Lateral Raises
3-4 x 12-15
Front Lateral Raises
3-4 x 12-15
Bent Lateral Raises
3-4 x 12-15
AB EXERCISES - Crunches
4 x 25

Routine # 3
6 Day program Chest, Shoulders, Arms, Back, Legs and Abs – change exercises each day

(2 Exercises per body part – there is only one listed here – you need to add the other)

Monday
CHEST - Incline Dumbbell Presses
1 set x 15 reps
2-3 sets x 10 reps

Tuesday
SHOULDER TRAINING – Military Press
3-4 x 12-15

Wednesday
BICEPS - Standing Barbell Curls
3 x 15
TRICEPS - Lying Overhead Triceps Extensions
4-6 x 15
FOREARM & WRIST – Reverse curls
3 x 15

Thursday
BACK MUSCLES - One-Arm Dumbbell Rows
3 sets x 12-15 reps

Friday
LEG MUSCLES - Leg Presses
4-8 x 8-15
Lying Leg Curls
3-6 x 8-10
Seated Calf Raises
3-4 x 12

Saturday
AB EXERCISES - Crunches
4 x 25

CPSIA information can be obtained at www.ICGtesting.com
Printed in the USA
LVOW012124120613

338272LV00024B/773/P